COPING SUCCESSFULLY WITH PERIOD PROBLEMS

MARY-CLAIRE MASON is a freelance journalist with a special interest in health, who has written widely for national newspapers and magazines. She is the author of *Coping with Fibroids*, *Sexually Transmitted Infections*, and co-author of *Rheumatoid Arthritis – Your Medication Explained*, all published by Sheldon Press. Mary-Claire has contributed regularly to the health pages of *Bella*, the women's weekly magazine, for over ten years.

Overcoming Common Problems Series

Selected titles
A full list of titles is available from Sheldon Press,
36 Causton Street, London SW1P 4ST, and on our website at
www.sheldonpress.co.uk

Overcoming Common Problems Series

Overcoming Common Problems Series

Overcoming Common Problems

Coping Successfully with Period Problems

Mary-Claire Mason

sheldon **PRESS**

First published in Great Britain in 2005
Sheldon Press
36 Causton Street
London SW1P 4ST

British Library Cataloguing-in-Publication Data

A catalogue record for this book is available from the British Library

ISBN 0–85969–948–X

Typeset by Deltatype Limited, Birkenhead, Merseyside
Printed in Great Britain by
Ashford Colour Press

Contents

Acknowledgements

I'd like to thank the women, doctors and therapists who helped me with my research and, in particular, consultant gynaecologist Peter Bowen-Simpkins, who patiently and expertly went through lots of queries with me.

1
The normal period

When it comes to knowing whether or not you've got a problem with your periods, it's important to understand what's considered normal. However, as Catherine's story illustrates, this isn't always easy to determine.

My periods began when I was 14, which was quite late in my family. My sisters started having periods when they were about 12 so my mum was a bit worried when mine didn't start then, and she was relieved when they did arrive. I just had the occasional one to start with. I didn't find them painful, but I did bleed a lot and I remember once having to lie down because I was passing so many clots.

I went on the Pill from about 18 to 25, which was great as I had no period problems, just relatively painless bleeds, but I had to come off the Pill because my blood pressure started to go up. After that my periods became heavy and painful, though they were always regular. I just coped as best I could. I wore double protection – tampons and pads together – and, even so, remember having an embarrassing accident at a friend's flat. I was sitting down and suddenly felt wet after a great gush of blood came out of me. I stood up and looked down at the sofa and saw a large red stain there. My friend was so kind, but I felt mortified.

I used to dread the first few hours before my period because I had a lot of pain, which was like a tight fist in my stomach. Several times I remember having to take a hot water bottle with me to work to cope with the pain. Somehow I managed to cope with the hot water bottle and painkillers, and I never took time off work. What really helped was Nurofen. My doctor advised me to take this for another problem. I read on the packet that you could also take it for period pain, so I tried it, and it was wonderful. Previously I'd tried other painkillers, such as paracetamol, but they weren't that effective, and Feminax just gave me a dry mouth. The good thing was that, once the bleeding got underway, the pain went.

From my late thirties onwards, my periods started to become

1

more erratic. I'd previously had a cycle of around 26 days, but that changed to 22, 23 24, 20, then up to 36, 38, back to 26, 40 and so on. They were all over the place and then started to get even more chaotic as I got near the menopause – for instance, 27, 77, 30, 31, 47, 21, 121. They became less painful, but I became anaemic because of the heavy bleeding at one point. I also started to spot several days before my periods began, which worried me, but I never saw the doctor about this and just hoped it was nothing to worry about.

I realized that I was approaching the menopause because I started to have hot flushes, so I had a blood test, which confirmed that I was menopausal. I had my last period when I was 49, which was 6 years ago.

I never really thought about whether I had problem periods or not. They were difficult to manage and I had to use lots of sanitary protection and they were also painful, but I just put up with the problems and used to dread the start of my periods. The spotting did worry me, but that became normal for me. I think that's an important point. My periods changed as I got older, but I adjusted to them and they were normal for me, even though, looking back now, I can see that maybe they weren't. Also, at the back of my mind, I think I thought that my doctor wouldn't be able to offer me much help anyway, other than a hysterectomy, so I just struggled on. I didn't think about how my diet and lifestyle might affect my periods.

Like Catherine, many women worry about their periods at some point in their lives. Painful and heavy periods can make life a misery, and periods usually change in some way or another over a woman's reproductive life, which can seem very worrying. The good news is that now more is known about periods, why problems occur and what can be done about them. There are more treatments on offer and there are many simple steps you can take yourself to solve problems.

The scale of period problems

Around 15 million women in this country are likely to be having periods because they're aged between 14 and 50 – the time span known as the childbearing years. Women have far more periods nowadays than they used to – in fact, around ten times more – which makes it more likely that you'll experience problems at some point or other. It's estimated that the average woman has around 400 periods in her lifetime, which means that we spend around 6 years having periods. In the past, when there was no contraception and women were pregnant more frequently and breastfeeding for longer, it's estimated that each woman had around 40 periods in her lifetime.

Everyone knows that women can have problems with periods, which explains why a common term for a period is 'the curse'. The amount of suffering women undergo was highlighted in a study in 2004. A total of 1500 women were asked about their reproductive health in the study, which was commissioned by WOW (Wellbeing of Women) – a charity that funds research into women's health. The researchers found that 50 per cent of the women had experienced problems such as heavy, irregular or painful periods or PMS in the past few years and some had had a mix of problems. Younger women were most likely to see their doctor about heavy periods and unusual bleeding, those between 36 and 45 about heavy periods and PMS and older women about menopausal symptoms. As a result of their monthly cycles, women felt less well for around 3.4 days a month and some women felt ill for as many as 10 days a month.

What is a period?

Menstruation, the bleeding commonly known as a period, is the outward sign of the monthly (menstrual) cycle and takes place at the start of the cycle. It's a process in which the womb lining is shed if no pregnancy has occurred in the previous cycle.

The purpose of the cycle, which is governed by a delicate balance of various hormones, is to release a mature egg. Once it has been fertilized by a sperm, the egg then implants in the lining of the womb, which is able to support the developing embryo.

A baby girl is born with about 2 million eggs, but, by the time she starts having periods – known as the menarche, which occurs in puberty – only about 300,000 eggs remain, as many shrivel and die in the intervening years between birth and puberty.

The length of the monthly cycle is counted from the first day of menstrual bleeding through to the last day before the next period starts.

The age at which periods first start occurs earlier than it used to –

3

on average at around 12.5 years whereas it was around 17 years 150 years ago. Girls' periods are starting at an earlier age due to a better diet. Girls need to weigh around 47 kg (a little under $7\frac{1}{2}$ stone) before periods start, but, if they haven't started by around 15 years, it's a good idea to see a doctor. It's unlikely that there is anything seriously wrong, but it makes sense to get medical advice, just in case there's some underlying cause for the lack of periods.

The next milestone is when your periods end. Women often talk loosely about the menopause as though it's a long period of change. In fact, strictly speaking, the run-up to the menopause is called the perimenopause and the menopause is actually the last period you have. Generally women have their last period between 45 and 55, with the average age being 50. However, some women can go through a much earlier menopause, known as a premature menopause – usually defined as occurring before 40. A tendency to early menopause may run in the family or be triggered by, for instance, cancer treatments, smoking or hysterectomy. The Daisy Network is a support group for women who've gone through a premature menopause (see Chapter 10 for contact details).

How the monthly cycle works

A complex balance of hormones governs the monthly cycle and ensures that a mature egg is produced and the lining of the womb is able to support a fertilized egg. A communication system between the brain and the ovaries allows this to happen. The following is a simple description of what is in fact a highly sophisticated process. The hypothalamus in the brain (which has various functions, including coordinating hormone systems in the body) sends GnRH (gonadotrophin releasing hormone) to the pituitary gland (hormonal control centre), also in the brain, to get it to produce two hormones known as gonadotrophins – FSH (follicle stimulating hormone) and LH (luteinizing hormone). These two hormones stimulate the ovaries to produce the hormones oestrogen (the ovaries produce oestradiol, the most powerful form of oestrogen) and progesterone.

Oestrogen has various jobs to do, including getting the eggs to ripen and the womb lining to grow. Progesterone – known often as the pregnancy hormone – has several functions, including the important one of thickening the womb lining ready for pregnancy.

At the start of each cycle, in response to low levels of oestrogen

4

and progesterone, the pituitary gland produces FSH – a signal to the ovaries to start the egg-ripening process. The follicles are lined with cells that produce oestrogen, which make the lining of the womb grow.

There are two parts to the monthly cycle. The first part is known as the follicular or proliferative phase. Egg follicles (blister-like structures containing eggs) are stimulated, but only one should develop and ripen into a mature egg. It's released at ovulation in response to a surge in LH, which is due to rising levels of inhibin – a substance produced by the follicle.

The second part of the cycle – known as the luteal or secretory phase – occurs after the egg is released at ovulation. The corpus luteum develops in the remains of the follicle and makes oestrogen and, especially, progesterone, which helps to make the lining of the womb richer and able to sustain an embryo, should one implant into it. If no fertilized egg implants into the lining, oestrogen and progesterone levels fall, there is less blood flow to the womb, so the lining starts to break down and is shed, together with blood, as a period at the start of the next monthly cycle.

Cycle length and regular cycles

The classic length is defined as 28 days – 14 days for the first part and 14 for the second part of the cycle – but women can have naturally longer or shorter cycles than this that are perfectly normal and nothing to worry about. The odd erratic cycle that doesn't fit into the normal pattern is also usually nothing to be worried about.

Gynaecologists give slightly differing figures for what is a normal-length period – 25–35 days is most often quoted, but 21–35 is given by some and even 21–42. Taking the longer period length, a cycle of, say, 40 days would be defined as regular. Whichever of these figures is quoted to you, if your cycle is under 21 days or over 42 days you'll be told that you have irregular periods.

The cycle is also described as irregular if it varies by more than about a couple of days either side of its usual length. If it's inside the normal definition, but swings from, say, 25 days one month to 38 and then down to 27 and so on, that would be considered irregular.

When calculating what's going on, it's also useful to know that the luteal phase (the second half of the cycle after ovulation) is fixed in terms of length at about 14 days. It's the follicular phase that varies in length. In a cycle of, say, 40 days, it's the first part of the cycle that is longer than average, at 26 days.

Regular cycles are normally a sign that you're ovulating and irregular ones that you're not ovulating regularly.

Anovulatory (eggless) cycles

In some cycles, no egg is released, there is no corpus luteum, no luteal phase and progesterone levels don't increase. These sorts of cycles aren't usually that painful, may be heavy and are common in girls who are starting to have periods and women coming up to the menopause.

The reason for this is that a balance of hormones is needed to ensure a normal ovulatory cycle, but hormones are often unbalanced at the start and towards the end of a woman's childbearing years.

Normal blood loss

When the old womb lining breaks down, it is shed along with blood as a period. Around 35–40 ml is a tight definition of what's defined as normal loss (around 2–3 tablespoons), but a looser, perhaps more realistic, one is 10–100 ml, though textbooks all define 80 ml and over as heavy bleeding (see Chapter 3 for more on this subject). Around 22 tampons or pads are used during an average period. A normal-length period is defined as around two to six days, with the heaviest bleeding on the first two or three days and this then tapers off.

Scanty, very light periods are fine if your periods have always been like that, but normal blood loss that changes to light blood loss could indicate ovulatory problems and possibly ovarian failure. This is a sign of some underlying condition, such as a thyroid abnormality, or could be the result of severe weight loss. Scanty periods that become heavier could be a sign of hormonal imbalance or fibroids or some other condition. (Heavy periods are looked at in detail in Chapter 3.)

Are periods important?

Periods are an outward sign of fertility and important if you want to have children, but, if you don't want them, do you still need to have periods? There's an argument that women can have too many periods and that repeated ovarian stimulation during each monthly cycle may increase the risk of ovarian cancer developing later in life. That's why women who have had children are thought to have a lower risk of developing the disease because they've had fewer cycles than women who have not had children.

Shedding the womb lining every so often, however, if not necessarily each month, is important as the risk of cancer of the lining of the womb increases if it builds up too much. The monthly production of oestrogen is also important, especially in younger women, for establishing strong bones. This reduces the risk of the bone-thinning disease, osteoporosis, developing in later life.

Should you worry if periods change?

It's very common for periods to change for all sorts of reasons (see below) and this is quite normal. If you have the occasional period that is different in some way from your usual period, don't panic. It's most likely the result of hormonal disturbance due, for instance, to stress. If you've been having periods and they then stop, allow up to six months for them to return. If they don't and you're not pregnant, then take medical advice. The chances are that nothing is wrong, but periods could have stopped due to a pituitary tumour, though this is rare, or some other sort of problem, such as a thyroid disorder. (For other reasons, see also under the heading What affects the monthly cycle?, below.)

Withdrawal bleeds

Women who are on the combined Pill have a monthly bleed, but this is not a period because there's no monthly cycle and no ovulation. When you take the Pill, the pituitary gland stops producing FSH because of the higher levels of oestrogen in the body from the Pill, so there's no ovulation.

The combination of oestrogen and progestogen (a synthetic version of the natural hormone progesterone) taken for 21 days keeps the womb lining thin. A withdrawal bleed occurs in the following seven-day pill-free week.

Strictly speaking, there's no need for this bleed because the lining is thin anyway. The argument was that women would want to have a bleed each month, though some doctors argue that it's important to have a pill-free week each month to allow blood fats to normalize and so reduce the risk of clots developing. Sometimes Pill packs are run together for up to three months if it makes sense not to have a bleed for some reason (see Chapter 6 on PMS). If you run the packs together for longer, you can get breakthrough bleeding in the Pill cycle, and that's a nuisance. If you don't have a bleed, it's usually nothing to worry about, though, of course, if you haven't taken the pills correctly you may be pregnant.

What affects the monthly cycle?

All sorts of things can disrupt the complex balance of hormones that rule the menstrual cycle. The result may be amenorrhoea, which means no periods, irregular periods, heavy periods or a range of other problems.

- *Stress* can temporarily disrupt cycles and is a likely reason for the very short cycle mentioned earlier on. The importance of stress can't be overestimated – it's a thread that runs throughout this book and is implicated in all period problems. You could say that the amount of stress in your life is reflected in your periods!
- *Crash dieting and becoming underweight* can send hormones haywire. If body fat falls below around 17 per cent, periods will stop.
- *Overweight women* may also stop ovulating. Women who carry more fat produce more oestrogen and too much oestrogen means that the brain may stop producing the hormones that cause ovulation.
- *Overexercising* can also result in a lack of periods.
- *Diseases and illnesses* can cause problems. For example, thyroid disorders (the thyroid gland is one of the main hormone glands in the body and regulates energy), such as an overactive or underactive thyroid, can cause irregular periods or heavy ones or anovulatory cycles. Women who have lupus – an autoimmune disorder in which the body's immune system attacks the body – may have period problems. Liver and kidney disease can also affect periods. Poorly controlled asthma may switch off the menstrual cycle.

- *Smoking* may cause more painful or heavier periods or irregular cycles.
- *Medicines* taken for other conditions may have an effect. For instance, if you take a steroid called prednisolone for a long time, you may find that your periods stop. Antidepressants called selective serotonin reuptake inhibitors, such as Prozac, may occasionally make periods a bit more painful. Drugs taken for manic depression, such as chloropromazine, may also stop periods. Two blood pressure medicines – spironolactone and methyldopa – can cause erratic bleeding. Spironolactone also has anti-masculinizing effects and is sometimes used to treat acne and excess body hair in women who have PCOS (polycystic ovary syndrome). Tamoxifen – the anti-oestrogen drug used for breast cancer treatment and sometimes for breast pain – can make cycles a bit irregular.

  Sodium valproate – a drug used to control epileptic seizures – may be linked to the development of PCOS, though there's a debate about whether it's the drug or epilepsy that makes women with epilepsy more prone to PCOS. Chemotherapy treatment for cancer stops ovulation. Some herbs taken on a long-term basis may also affect the cycle. For example, the stress-busting herb ginseng, if taken for more than three months, may make periods irregular. Before you start any long-term medication, ask if it affects the menstrual cycle and, if it does, whether there are any alternatives or if it can be used in a lower dose to minimize problems. If you've started to take some medication and you notice a change in your monthly cycle, ask your doctor or pharmacist or therapist if this could be due to the medication. It's always a case of weighing up the pros and cons of each medicine when treating a condition.
- *Childbirth* is often said to result in less painful periods afterwards. The reason for this is that menstrual blood is squeezed out of the womb through the os, which is a small opening in the cervix. After a vaginal birth, the opening is larger, so, for some women, periods may become less painful.
- *Around the menopause* cycles may go haywire as hormone levels fluctuate. Sometimes cycles may become very short or long and irregular, periods may stop or get very heavy and then everything may return to normal for a time.
- *The stress of travelling* can upset the monthly cycle.

- *Sterilization* Some women say that their periods get heavier after sterilization. There's no reason for this, say most gynaecologists, and modern sterilization techniques are less invasive. What's probably happening is that women are getting used to having natural periods again. For instance, if they were on the Pill before they were sterilized, they would have had light withdrawal bleeds, but see Sue's experience in Chapter 3 on heavy periods.
- *Contraception* The coil can make periods heavier and more painful than normal (see Chapter 2 for more on IUDs).

The menstrual cycle and other conditions

It's important to be aware of the monthly cycle's effects on other conditions. For instance, about one in three women who suffer from asthma find that their symptoms get worse around the time of their period, especially if they suffer from severe asthma. The hormones oestrogen and progesterone have an anti-inflammatory effect, but levels of these hormones drop before a period, so there's less protection from attacks.

Some migraine sufferers get menstrual migraine, which is when attacks occur around the time of their period due to falling levels of oestrogen. Some women who have epilepsy find that they have more seizures around the time of their period because oestrogen levels, though falling, are higher than progesterone levels at that point – oestrogen can provoke seizures while progesterone has the opposite effect.

Some women say that their irritable bowel syndrome symptoms worsen premenstrually. There's also some research that suggests that rheumatoid arthritis symptoms may not be so bad during the second part of the cycle. Women who have diabetes may find it harder to control blood sugar levels at certain points in their cycle and the autoimmune condition lupus can flare up premenstrually.

Delaying periods and stopping withdrawal bleeds

Most women on the combined Pill are on the monophasic type, which means that each tablet contains the same amount of hormones in it. If you're on this type of Pill, it's possible, as previously discussed, to run pill packs together for up to three months so that you won't have a withdrawal bleed. There isn't usually a problem with doing this, but double-check with your doctor that it's safe for you to do, for example, if you don't want to have a bleed because you're going travelling. Biphasic or triphasic pills contain different amounts of hormones so you won't be able to run pill packs together.

If you're not on the Pill and want to delay your period, progestogen can be prescribed. Once you stop taking it, the womb lining starts to break down and you have a period in about 48 hours. It's usually safe to postpone bleeding in this way for a couple of months, but not a good idea to do it for longer because progestogen may affect heart health by causing the formation of fatty substances, which can damage blood vessels. Progestogen also has side-effects such as bloating and mood swings.

Key points

There's no hard and fast definition of what a normal period is, though there is some general guidance, as we've seen, and that's important to know. What is clearly 'normal' is for periods to change in some way or other at various points during your childbearing years.

2
Period pain

While there are the lucky few who will sail through their periods pain free, period pain is a fact of life for most women. Perhaps as many as eight out of ten will have pain for some, if not most, of their periods. Around 10 per cent of women are so affected each month that they can't carry on as normal and have to take time off because the pain leaves them doubled up in agony.

What causes the pain?

The womb contracts during menstruation to get rid of the old lining of the womb, so that a new one can form for the next cycle. There are various explanations as to why the pain happens during this shedding process. As the contractions take place, blood supply to the womb is reduced as the blood vessels are squeezed. This means that tissue may not get enough oxygen and that can result in pain.

The discomfort occurs in cycles in which ovulation takes place. There's speculation that the pain may be linked in some way to the increased production of progesterone, which happens in the second half of these cycles. In contrast, anovulatory cycles are usually much less painful and that may be because there's no increase in progesterone as no egg has been released.

The role of progesterone in pain is unclear, but what is certain is that prostaglandins play an important part in the pain. There are various types of prostaglandins – natural hormone-like chemicals produced in the body that have various functions. Though some are beneficial and have an anti-inflammatory effect in the body, others have an inflammatory effect, encourage period cramps and reduce blood flow to the womb. They are thus an important cause of symptoms such as painful spasms, diarrhoea, vomiting and nausea. Women who experience much pain may produce a lot of these chemicals and/or be particularly sensitive to them.

As explained in the last chapter, pain may also occur when menstrual blood and clots pass through the small opening in the neck of the womb called the cervical os. After a vaginal birth, some

12

women find that their periods are less painful and this may be because the os has been stretched during labour.

To add to all this, stress, anxiety and worry make period pain worse.

Primary dysmenorrhoea

The medical name for period pain is dysmenorrhoea and there are two types – primary and secondary. Primary dysmenorrhoea usually starts once the monthly cycle has established itself and ovulation has begun in the teenage years, so it may take a couple of years or so before teenagers start to get painful periods.

The acute symptoms of primary spasmodic dysmenorrhoea include painful cramps in the lower abdomen (similar to the pain of contractions in childbirth), vomiting, feeling faint and backache. The discomfort usually starts a few hours before bleeding, but the worst of it is normally over as bleeding gets underway. The symptoms may last anything from around 4 to 24 hours, but usually less than 12 hours.

On top of having to cope with these acute symptoms, some women also have what's called congestive dysmenorrhoea, which can occur before a period starts. Symptoms include an aching, heavy sensation in the pelvis, feeling tired, bloated, clumsy and emotionally very sensitive – PMS-type symptoms. This chapter is about the spasmodic pain, but following the advice in Chapter 6 on PMS and the section on self-help and lifestyle later in this chapter should help relieve the congestive symptoms as well.

Secondary dysmenorrhoea

This is the name used when underlying conditions cause period pain. Examples of such conditions include endometriosis – where the womb lining escapes into the pelvic cavity (see the section on this condition at the end of this chapter) – fibroids, non-cancerous lumps in the womb wall, pelvic inflammatory disease (the result of untreated sexually transmitted infections, which can cause a host of problems including increased period pain, see below for more on this subject). Another is adenomyosis, which is when deposits from the womb lining get into the muscular womb wall. Adenomyosis is a

13

little-understood condition and can be confused with fibroids. It tends to affect women in their forties and may cause pain throughout the period (there is some more information on this condition after the section on endometriosis at the end of this chapter).

Irritable bowel syndrome (IBS)

IBS is a really common condition characterized by a collection of symptoms that include diarrhoea, constipation, bloating and abdominal pain. The symptoms are real, but it's called a functional disorder because there are no apparent signs of disease or other abnormalities in the gut. Some women who have this condition get painful periods, too – possibly because the pelvic area is more sensitive than normal as a result of having IBS.

If you suffer from painful periods and have IBS symptoms, it's worth asking your doctor if IBS could be the reason for your pain, to prevent the pain being misdiagnosed as a gynaecological problem. For more information on IBS, contact the IBS Network (see Chapter 10).

Is period pain serious?

No, not usually if it's the primary sort, but that doesn't mean you should put up with it! If simple treatments don't help, it's a good idea to talk to your doctor about stronger treatments if the pain is interfering with your everyday life. It's also important to see your GP to rule out other problems. If the pain pattern changes or you get pain at other times of the month, this could be a sign of some underlying condition that needs to be sorted out.

- Keep a diary to identify when you're getting pain.
- Pain that lasts throughout your period, is getting worse or starts several days before your period plus painful sex could mean endometriosis (see the section on this condition near the end of this chapter).
- Pelvic congestion is another condition that can cause abdominal discomfort at other times of the month. If your pelvis aches after exercise or when you've been standing for a long time, for example, this could be a sign of pelvic congestion, thought to be a

stress-related condition. The ovaries produce too much oestrogen, resulting in blood pooling in slack pelvic veins.

• If you're getting clots, heavy and painful periods and/or your stomach is expanding, you may have fibroids. One-sided pain and a swollen abdomen could be a sign of an ovarian cyst. There are various types of ovarian cysts. Often they cause no problems, but, depending on the type and position, may cause abdominal discomfort, painful sex or make periods irregular. Cysts may sometimes have to be removed and emergency surgery may be needed if a cyst suddenly twists, causing acute pain. The Pill is sometimes prescribed to stop cysts forming.

• Any sudden, severe pain on one side needs to be investigated as it may be a sign of an ectopic pregnancy or a ruptured cyst.

Pelvic inflammatory disease (PID)

It's important to get medical advice if you have PID. It occurs as the result of an untreated sexually transmitted infection moving into the pelvis.

It's a potentially serious infection that can cause a lot of pain and result in infertility. Symptoms can include tiredness, heavy and painful periods, bleeding in between periods and an abnormal vaginal discharge. Don't ignore these symptoms; it's important to go to a sexual health clinic to be tested.

Intrauterine devices (IUDs)

If you're thinking about having an IUD contraceptive fitted, check with your doctor whether or not this is a good idea.

An IUD is a small plastic and copper device that is fitted inside the womb to prevent conception. IUDs work very well and many women are happy with them but perhaps as many as half find that their periods become more painful and heavier as a result of having an IUD fitted.

If you already suffer from period pain, ask if it's a good idea to have one fitted. If you decide on one, try to make sure that it's fitted by someone who is skilled in fitting them. Those who insert just one a year are not likely to be as skilled as those who regularly fit them. Discuss also whether you want to continue with one if your periods become painful after insertion. Also, if you develop a high temperature and pain in the abdomen in the first three weeks after your IUD has been inserted, see your doctor because you could have an infection. Ideally, you should be screened for sexually transmitted infections before having one inserted.

There are different types of IUDs. The shape and size of your womb should be measured to find out, first of all, whether or not an IUD can be fitted and then to assess which one would be best for you. Women who have had children are unlikely to have more painful periods afterwards, provided the IUD is fitted correctly. Women who haven't had children may have more problems because their wombs haven't been stretched by pregnancy and pain may occur when the womb squeezes the rigid plastic frame of the IUD. However, there's now a flexible IUD – Gynefix – that consists of several small copper beads threaded on to a length of nylon. This may be a better bet if you've got a smaller womb because then there's nothing for the womb to squeeze on.

Getting rid of period pain

Steps can be taken just before and during your period to stop the pain. Lifestyle measures such as altering your diet and controlling levels of stress throughout the month can help enormously.

The good news is that there are now lots of treatment options available – from the simple to the more complicated. What you choose will depend on whether or not you want to become pregnant. For example, taking the Pill (discussed below) is an effective treatment, but this option obviously isn't any good if you're trying to conceive or are unable to take it.

Non-prescription treatments

The following simple treatments do not affect fertility and can be taken just around the time of your period.

Vitamin E supplement

This option may be worth trying before anything else as a new study found that taking a vitamin E supplement significantly reduced period pain and also cut blood loss, though, of course, more research needs to be done to confirm these results. In the study, reported in the *British Journal of Obstetrics and Gynaecology* (April 2005, vol. 112, pp. 466–9), 278 girls aged 15–17 who suffered from varying degrees of period pain were split into two groups. One group took vitamin E tablets and the other group a placebo (dummy pill). In the vitamin E group, the girls took 200 IU vitamin E twice a day (a 400 IU daily dose, which is the equivalent of a 200-mg dose say the researchers) for five days – two days before the period and then for the first three days of bleeding – for four months. Those in the vitamin E group had significantly less pain and less bleeding than those in the placebo group. The pain relief experienced was greatest for those who had severe period pain.

Vitamin E is reported to work by reducing prostaglandin production. A bonus is that it's thought to be relatively free of side-effects. If you've had clots, though, check with your doctor whether or not it's safe for you to take.

Painkillers can be taken with the vitamin E tablets if you have pain. If you decide to try vitamin E, make sure that you take it two days before your period starts (as happened in the study) as this helps to cut down prostaglandin production. Try it for several periods to see if it helps.

Non-steroidal anti-inflammatory drugs (NSAIDs)

These include ibuprofen, of which there are many brands such as Nurofen and Librofem. These are probably the best painkillers to start with. They also work by blocking production of the prostaglandins that cause pain. Aspirin is a similar sort of drug.

As with all drugs, NSAIDs can have a range of side-effects, including nausea, vomiting and stomach pain, and they're unsuitable if you've suffered from stomach ulcers or have asthma.

Don't wait for the pain to start – take the drug sooner rather than later so that you nip pain in the bud. Start it as soon as you have the slightest symptom or twinge. Some gynaecologists advise beginning the medicine a day or two before your period starts to block the build-up of prostaglandins. If you have irregular periods, however, it's more difficult to do this unless you can detect the early warning signs of an approaching period. Continue to take the tablets and don't stop when the pain starts to ease a bit.

Other options

If NSAIDs don't work for you or you can't take them because you have asthma or stomach problems, there are other options (and see the section on vitamin E above).

Painkillers – or analgesics as they're called – can be very effective for combatting period pain. Take advice from a pharmacist about what's available in order to find one that suits you. Non-opioid pills, such as paracetamol, work by stopping the transmission of pain in that part of the body where you're getting pain. Opioids such as codeine are related to opium and work on the brain to alter your perception of pain. They are used in combination with other analgesics.

Always check what's in a product, as some of them may contain several ingredients – codeine, paracetamol and so on – as well as caffeine.

Codeine may cause constipation, which can make period pain worse. Caffeine may cause insomnia, headaches and nausea in those sensitive to it. Paracetamol is safe on the stomach, but can cause liver and kidney damage and may prove fatal if overdosing occurs. So, as with any medicine, always check and follow the safety instructions.

Feminax – designed specifically for period pain – contains caffeine, paracetamol and codeine, as well as hyoscine, which is a muscle relaxant to ease cramps, but it may cause a dry mouth.

Prescription treatments

A range of other drugs can be prescribed by doctors if you find that the non-prescription pills don't work. Most of these options are contraceptives, however, and affect your body throughout the month. Clearly they will not be suitable if you want to become pregnant or don't want to or can't take hormonal treatments.

Stronger NSAIDS

These need to be prescribed. They can be taken when you have pain and won't affect your fertility. Mefenamic acid (Ponstan) is the best-known medicine in this group of drugs for period pain and usually you will need to take a 500-mg tablet three times a day. It's safest taken after food, to avoid stomach irritation.

There are other drugs in this group, such as naproxen. If you can't keep the medicine down because of vomiting, it's worth asking if an NSAID can be prescribed as a suppository rather than as a tablet – a diclofenac suppository, for example. This can be a highly effective way of taking such medicine.

As with the non-prescription NSAIDs, gynaecologists say that these medicines work best if you start them the day before bleeding starts. This is fine if you have regular cycles, but many women don't, so it may not always be possible to do this.

The combined pill

This treatment works very well for problems like painful periods. The two hormones in the Pill keep the womb lining very thin so that the resulting withdrawal bleed is usually light, short and much less painful. There's no ovulation, so no natural period occurs.

A monophasic preparation is the one most often taken and gives you the same amount of oestrogen and progestogen each day for 21 days, followed by a 7-day break. There are around 17 brands and they're not identical to each other in terms of dosage and make-up, so there's some choice. Yasmin, for instance, is a newer Pill that has a type of progestogen in it that is claimed to help relieve the uncomfortable feeling of fluid retention some women experience with some of the older progestogen formulations. So, if possible, try to explore the options.

It is important, too, to weigh up the pros and cons of taking the Pill with your doctor. If, for instance, you suffer from severe migraine or have had blood clots in the past or smoke and are 35 or older, then the Pill may not be suitable for you. Women also have a slightly increased risk of developing breast cancer if they've been on the Pill, but research shows that this risk disappears ten years after stopping the Pill. If you're trying for a baby then obviously the Pill isn't an option for you and nor is it for women who don't want to use hormonal treatments.

Mirena intrauterine system (IUS)

This is a device that is fitted inside the womb that acts by releasing a type of progestogen called levonorgestrel. It's a contraceptive that works by keeping the womb lining so thin that an embryo can't implant in it. It also thickens cervical mucus so that sperm can't get into the womb and it suppresses ovulation sometimes, though most women with the Mirena do still ovulate.

As a result of having such a thin lining, many women end up having very light periods (after a year there's a big reduction in blood loss) or none at all (one in five women stop having periods a year after the Mirena has been inserted), so the device has been licensed as a treatment for heavy periods.

It may reduce painful periods, too, because it reduces the amount of flow. In one study of 50 women given the Mirena for heavy periods, not only was blood loss substantially reduced – by about 80 per cent – but also they experienced less pain.

The Mirena lasts for up to five years and, once it's removed, fertility returns. It should have no detrimental effect on bone health and, because the progestogen works where it's needed, in the womb, there are far fewer side-effects than taking progestogen as a tablet treatment.

It does have some disadvantages, however. Many women, for instance, have breakthrough bleeding and spotting for the first few months, but this usually settles down. In addition, the Mirena can sometimes be expelled from the womb. The Mirena is also a bit wider than conventional IUDs and women who've never given birth vaginally may find the fitting a bit more painful than those who have done so. The solution is to have a local anaesthetic when the Mirena is inserted.

Heavy and painful periods

As many women know all too well, painful and heavy periods often go hand in hand – it's not a question of one or the other, though it may be for some women. The combined Pill is a good treatment for both heavy and painful periods, the Mirena is an excellent treatment for heavy periods and may well reduce pain, too, as we've just seen, and, clearly, if you stop having periods, you won't have pain!

Doctors can also prescribe mefenamic acid (Ponstan) – one of the stronger NSAIDs mentioned briefly above. This stops not only pain but also bleeding (see Chapter 3). Ponstan can be prescribed together with tranexamic acid (Cyklokapron – also discussed in Chapter 3). There are no cross-reactions between the two drugs, but it does mean that you have to take a lot of tablets each day! On the other hand, these drugs don't affect fertility and need only be taken during your period so it's worth asking your doctor about this option if you don't want to take long-term hormonal treatments.

Self-help and lifestyle

Apart from medicines, there are lots of things you can do yourself to ease the pain. First, treat the pain itself and, second, take measures throughout the month that help to make periods less painful.

A hot water bottle

This is a simple, but highly effective, way of easing the muscular contractions that can cause discomfort. The heat relaxes the muscles and gets the blood flowing again, which stops the pain.

Try putting one on your lower abdomen and maybe another one in the small of your back – do whatever gives you the most comfort. Lie quietly with one or two bottles in place and wait for the pain to ease.

The only problem is that hot water bottles are bulky and difficult to use if you're at work. However, there are more discreet thermal products that act like a hot water bottle and you could wear these to work – ask your pharmacist what's on offer.

Breathing

If you breathe slowly, low and deep down in the abdomen, this aids relaxation and stops the automatic response of breathing shallowly and tensing up that can occur if you're in pain.

Breathe in through your nose and then sigh and relax on the out-breath, taking longer to breathe out than in.

TENS

TENS stands for transcutaneous electrical nerve stimulation and is a way of triggering production of the body's natural chemical defences against pain – endorphins.

This is achieved by wearing a TENS machine, which sends out a small electrical pulse through electrodes attached to the skin and this stimulates the spinal nerves to produce endorphins that help to block pain messages.

It's used for pain relief in childbirth and there's good evidence that it works for period pain too. It's a drug-free, simple and safe method to use and can be worn under clothes (see Chapter 10 for contact details for a supplier).

Biolamp

This is another product that may ease pain and is thought to work by improving circulation in the pelvic area.

The Biolamp, when heated up, gives off electromagnetic waves released from 33 minerals implanted within a ceramic plate. It is claimed to be good for severe period pain and other pain. The lamp is shone on to the bare skin of the abdomen for 20 minutes of each

21

day of your period. Pat, who suffered from bad period pain, said, 'it felt like someone's hand taking away the pain. I was pain-free for the rest of the day'.

Acupressure

This is a drug-free method that is worth trying. Acupressure – a non-invasive technique derived from acupuncture – involves the application of pressure to certain points on the body using the fingers or thumbs.

More than nine out of ten college students said that it helped reduce period pain in a study in Taiwan, published in the *Journal of Advanced Nursing*. Pressure was applied to the Sanyinjiao point on the inside of the ankle for 20 minutes a day. Thirty-five students in the acupressure group were compared to women in a control group who didn't receive treatment. Study results showed that 94 per cent of the women in the group receiving treatment were moderately to extremely satisfied with the results. Students were then shown how to apply the technique themselves.

If you want to try, measure the width of four fingers above the ankle bone on the inside of your leg. To find the correct spot to press, slide your finger off the edge of the shinbone towards the inside of your leg – the area may feel a bit sensitive. Apply firm thumb pressure for six seconds, release for two seconds, then continue this pattern for five minutes. Do the same on the other ankle. Repeat this process until you've done it for 20 minutes.

Strong chamomile tea and other herbal remedies

This tea is well known as a relaxant and should help relieve womb cramps. Ginger tea improves circulation. Cramp bark (the guelder rose) calms the womb and is a good, safe remedy for period pain. It's available from healthfood shops as a tablet or in liquid form as a tincture.

Evening primrose oil

A 1000-mg dose taken daily throughout the cycle can significantly reduce bleeding and pain, according to one doctor.

Flower essence

She Oak may reduce painful cramps (see *Heal Yourself with Flowers and Other Essences* by Nikki Bradford (Quadrille, 2005).

Smoking

Smoking heightens pain by increasing contractions and reducing blood supply to the womb, so this is another reason to give up if you're a smoker.

Constipation

This can make period pain worse and often seems to happen just before a period, so it's a good idea to take steps to prevent it. Drink lots of fluid and eat plenty of fibre throughout the month to reduce the likelihood of getting constipated and avoid painkillers such as codeine, which can cause constipation.

Caffeine

It may make period cramps worse, according to some reports, and cutting it out may be the answer for some women. Lucy says, 'I used to drink a lot of strong black coffee every day, but, since I've stopped, my period pain has gone.' It's worth experimenting for a couple of months to see whether or not it helps you to cut right back on tea, coffee and fizzy drinks, such as cola, that contain caffeine.

Massage

This is a good, and enjoyable, option because it improves blood circulation.

Use firm, circular movements with your fingertips, working along the bikini line.

Yoga

With its emphasis on breathing and gentle stretching movements, yoga is good for general health as well as combating period pain.

There are some postures that are particularly good for period pain. Try sitting on the floor with a straight back, knees bent outwards with the soles of your feet together and rest your wrists on your knees. Stay in this position for several minutes and, as you breathe, think of tension flowing out of your body on each out-breath.

Susan Lark recommends several yoga postures for period pain in her book *Menstrual Cramps* (Celestial Arts, 1993). The Child pose is one of the most effective postures, she says. To do this, kneel on the floor, then sit back on your feet and lower your head to the floor in front of you, resting your forehead gently on the floor, and put your arms on the floor either side of you, pointing back towards your feet with the backs of your hands laying on the floor. Close your eyes and stay like this for as long as is comfortable.

Another posture is the Cat Cow, which practised regularly will prevent menstrual cramps and lower back pain. To get into position, kneel on all fours, then as you breathe in curve your spine downwards while lifting your eyes towards the ceiling so your head rolls up and back. Then, as you breathe out, round the spine up and lower your head down between your arms.

Diet

A diet that helps to keep oestrogen levels in check means a thinner womb lining and one that produces fewer prostaglandins. The result should be less painful periods. Neil Barnard, in his book *Foods That Fight Pain* (Bantam, 1999), tells how 19 women who suffered moderate to severe menstrual pain made changes to their diet. The women were asked to avoid animal products and eat simple, unprocessed foods, whole grains, vegetables and fruits. Most of the women noticed a change in their symptoms – they had a lot less pain or none at all, had more energy and lost weight.

There's nothing new about this sort of advice in terms of general health. We've known for a long time that eating whole foods and up to ten portions of fruit and vegetables a day, cutting back on fat, reducing meat consumption and eating fewer sugary foods, chocolate, cakes and biscuits is good for us, but it is good news that it's also likely to mean less period pain. The best thing is to try it and persevere for several months to see how your periods are affected.

B vitamins help the liver work more effectively, which means that it will clear out excess oestrogen in the body, says Dr Barnard. Try to eat plenty of wholegrain foods, beans, bananas and unsalted nuts, as these are good sources of vitamin B. Drinking too much alcohol can overload the liver and make it less able to get rid of excess oestrogen, so try to keep your alcohol consumption at a moderate to low level.

Omega 3 essential fatty acids have an anti-inflammatory action in the body, so eating foods rich in these is a good idea. The easiest way to boost omega 3 consumption is to eat oily fish, such as salmon, sardines and mackerel, but linseeds and pumpkin seeds are rich in these fatty acids, too.

Magnesium is a mineral that is responsible for, among other

24

things, nerve and muscle function and a deficiency of it has been linked to muscle cramps. There's also evidence that women don't get enough of this mineral and a lack of it could play a part in period cramps. It makes sense, then, to eat plenty of foods rich in magnesium and, if you follow the healthy eating advice above, you will as it's contained in green vegetables, nuts and whole grains – bananas are a particularly good source of it, as well as vitamin B. If you want to take a magnesium supplement, the recommended daily allowance for women is 270 mg. Make sure not to take more than 400 mg, as you may suffer diarrhoea and the long-term effects of taking high doses of magnesium are unknown, but there shouldn't be any harmful effects if you keep under that limit, says the Food Standards Agency.

Stress

It probably won't come as any surprise that stress makes periods more painful. According to a recent study, high levels of stress doubled the chances of suffering bad period pain. In the study, of the 388 women in China aged 20–34 who took part, only 22 per cent of those who reported low stress had painful periods, but 44 per cent of those who complained of high stress had painful periods.

If you think you're under a lot of stress, then it's important to get it under control. Destressing means discovering which parts of your life are causing stress and seeing what can be done about them. Regular exercise will help to burn off the stress hormones (see below and Chapter 7).

Exercise

It's accepted that we all lead too sedentary a life and that we need to exercise more in order to improve our general health. Vigorous exercise – exercising enough to get the heart pumping – eliminates stress hormones and increases production of endorphins, which, as we saw earlier, are the body's natural painkillers. All of this means that you'll feel better.

While it's accepted that women who exercise a lot have fewer period problems generally, there aren't currently any studies clearly showing that exercise eliminates period pain. However, logically, the benefits outlined above, the improved blood flow to the pelvis and the fact that the muscles are loosened up in the process should help.

25

Despite this, researchers, in a review of various studies that examined the relationship between exercise and period pain, concluded that there was no solid evidence to back up the claim that exercise helps period pain. What this means is that exercise may reduce period pain – it just hasn't been proved to do so at the moment. Another study concluded that, although exercise reduced stress, it might actually have aggravated pain symptoms. This, of course, calls into question how good the studies were, but also means that the link between aerobic exercise and period pain aren't clear at the moment. Thus, we can say from all this that, although regular aerobic exercise is beneficial for general health, it's not clear how helpful it is for period pain and that if you expect your pain to go just because you've taken up regular aerobic exercise, you may be disappointed (it certainly does help other period problems, however, as we'll see later in the book).

Exercise is important for all of us for a variety of other reasons – for heart health, bone strength and mental health – but you can over-exercise and that may prove counter-productive. So, when it comes to period pain, aim to do more vigorous exercise mid-cycle, but, around the time of your period, be guided by your body. Don't push yourself too hard – ease up and exercise more gently. Walking is ideal because you can use a faster pace earlier in the month but go at a slower pace around the time of your period and stop altogether if you feel unwell. The yoga positions outlined earlier should be helpful at such times. Do this and keep a note as to whether or not you have less pain as a result (see Chapter 9 for more on exercise).

Other therapies

Herbalism

Herbs can reduce pain and you can self-treat. Agnus castus tablets can be taken for two months to correct any hormonal imbalances in the body. Skullcap is a muscle relaxant that can be taken in tablet form during your period.

See a qualified herbalist if problems persist and for tailor-made help.

A word of warning: do approach taking herbs with caution – particularly if you think that you might be pregnant, have another condition, such as epilepsy, or are taking medication. Just because they are 'natural' doesn't mean that herbs have no side-effects and some herbs do interact with other substances. For example, St John's Wort should not be taken with the Pill, anti-epilepsy treatments and a number of other medications, including antidepressants, or with foods containing tyramine, such as cheese, red wine, preserved meats and yeast extracts. Do consult your doctor and take advice from a herbalist if in doubt or if you are taking any medication before you start taking herbs.

Homeopathy

In *The Women's Guide to Homeopathy* (Hamish Hamilton, 1992), Dr Andrew Lockie and Dr Nicola Geddes say that it's worth trying specific homeopathic remedies for period pain before you try anything else, such as painkillers from the pharmacy.

The remedy should be taken as soon as pain starts, in a 30 c (centesimal) dose every hour for up to 10 doses. The remedies include Belladonna 30 for when the pain is worse before the blood flow starts or when there's a dragging sensation. There are various other remedies, but the one that's best for you will depend on the mix of symptoms you have. As the 'remedy pictures' are quite detailed, it's probably best to see a qualified homeopath in order for the treatment to be most effective.

Acupuncture

Fine needles are inserted at various points to stimulate healing. It's widely used for a variety of conditions, but has a reputation for being good for pain relief.

In one study, acupuncture eased painful periods in over 90 per cent of women and there was a 40 per cent reduction in their use of painkillers.

Endometriosis

This section is devoted to a condition that is an important cause of bad period pain. A lot of women are affected by endometriosis – as many as 2 million women may have it, though it's difficult to know exactly how many as the only way to confirm a diagnosis is to look at the pelvic organs inside the abdomen.

Endometriosis is a mysterious condition in which cells from the womb lining get into the pelvic cavity where they attach themselves and bleed each month, causing inflammation, cysts and adhesions that may glue organs together. These cells can also get into the muscular wall of the womb, but a lot less is known about this condition, which is called adenomyosis (see below).

There are all sorts of ideas about why endometriosis occurs, but probably the one on which there is most agreement is that of retrograde menstruation. This term means that, during a period, bits of the womb lining that should flow out of the body instead flow back up through the Fallopian tubes and into the pelvis.

It's unclear what triggers endometriosis, though the condition seems to run in families, so some women have a genetic predisposition to developing it. There's also a theory that it's a 'modern woman's disease' – that the condition is more likely to develop in women now because we have far more periods now than we previously did.

Symptoms include severe period pain that doesn't respond to simple painkillers or bad pain for several days before bleeding starts, chronic pelvic pain throughout the cycle, deep pain during sex and it being painful when undergoing an internal examination. Opening the bowels or urinating may be painful, too, especially during periods.

Women suffering this condition can become infertile if the ovaries are badly affected or the Fallopian tubes are stuck down by the rogue tissue. Strangely, there's no link necessarily between the severity of symptoms and the amount of endometriosis in the pelvis. Some women have severe symptoms yet little endometrial tissue in the pelvis, while other women have extensive endometriosis in the pelvis but few symptoms.

The condition is diagnosed by doing a relatively minor keyhole operation called a laparoscopy, in which a couple of tiny punctures are made in the abdomen. The abdomen is then inflated with gas and a viewing instrument called a laparoscope is inserted to view the pelvic organs.

There has been research into establishing whether or not a magnetic resonance imaging (MRI) scan can help show up endometrial deposits in the pelvis. Some researchers are of the view that women with suspected endometriosis should have a laparoscopy and an MRI scan to reveal the true extent of endometriosis in the pelvis.

Treatment

What is appropriate for you depends on whether or not you want to become pregnant and the severity of your symptoms.

The combined pill

This is the first treatment of choice if you don't want to have a baby. Pill packs can be run together for up to three months to avoid having a bleed (under the supervision of a gynaecologist it may be possible to do this for longer).

Medication

A more complicated regime, but one that works well according to some gynaecologists, is to take a drug that puts you into a false state of menopause. This switches off the monthly production of hormones that fuel the disease. Drugs called gonadotrophin-releasing hormone (GnRH) analogues can be given to produce this effect, but you need a tiny amount of what's called 'addback' therapy to protect bone health and reduce menopausal symptoms if you're taking this for any length of time. Livial (tibolone) – a hormone replacement therapy (HRT) product – is often used for addback therapy. The benefits of this have to be balanced with the cons as there are safety concerns about HRT (see Chapter 10 for contact details of organizations that can provide more information).

Progestogen treatments, such as medroxyprogesterone, can be prescribed continuously to make you period-free, but they need to be taken in high doses to have this effect. There can be unpleasant side-effects, however, such as bloating, breast tenderness and mood swings.

Mirena IUS

This is being used by some gynaecologists to treat endometriosis, even though it's not yet licensed for this purpose. The argument is that it's a better way of providing progestogen than tablets as a much lower dose of progestogen is used in the Mirena because it works where it's needed, in the womb. The lower doses required mean that it causes far fewer side-effects than is the case for tablet treatment.

Many women stop having periods after several months with the Mirena, but it may also dry up diseased tissue in the pelvis, though it's not clear yet whether it can stop the disease progressing further.

A study published in the journal *Human Reproduction* (vol. 19, no. 1, pp. 179–84, January 2004) concluded that the Mirena worked well for mild to moderate endometriosis.

Sue, 36, has suffered from endometriosis since she was 20.

I've had six operations and all sorts of hormone treatments to switch off my cycle. A couple of years ago, my gynaecologist suggested the Mirena because I was having breakthrough bleeding with the Pill, so I had it inserted. Since then, I've had far fewer problems. The Mirena seems to have stabilized my condition and my symptoms haven't got worse. I get a bleed every six weeks, but it's so light it's not really like a period and I don't need to use sanitary protection.

I can still get some pain around the time of the bleeding, but it's not too bad – periods in the past used to be a dreadful ordeal because of the pain. The Mirena works well for me, though I've put on weight on my bottom as a result of it, but that's a small price to pay. It's a long-term treatment that I hope will see me through to the menopause, but I may have it out for a time and try for a baby as I've just got married. It's better than other treatments, which, because of their side-effects, can't be used long term.

What if you're trying for a baby?

The best option at the moment is to have surgery to remove endometrial deposits and, if that doesn't work, IVF treatment. However, in the pipeline, treatments include drugs called aromatase inhibitors, which have an anti-oestrogenic effect (used currently in the treatment of breast cancer) and selective oestrogen receptor modulators (SERMs), which may block the effect of oestrogen on the tissue lining the womb.

Endometriosis and diet

There's a lot of interest in whether or not some diets can help reduce the symptoms of endometriosis – particularly from women who've found that conventional approaches haven't been helpful. A study published in the journal *Human Reproduction* (vol. 19, no. 8, pp. 1755–9, July 2004), concluded that a diet rich in fruit and vegetables may cut the risk of endometriosis, while eating meat might increase the risk. It's only one study, but, if relatively simple dietary changes can make a difference, they are worth considering.

Ann, now in her mid thirties, was diagnosed with endometriosis in her mid twenties.

I got really heavy, painful periods and stomach ache throughout the month and ended up going to casualty, where endometriosis was diagnosed when a laparoscopy was done. I was put on some tablets that put me into a menopausal state, but I got dreadful symptoms. After I came off the drug, I was fine for a couple of years, but then my periods got really bad again, so I went on the Pill and also had surgery to burn away the deposits. The symptoms returned and I became very depressed because I was in so much pain and didn't know what to do.

I went to see a nutritionist who advised me to eat more fruit and veg and oily fish, and to cut back on fatty foods like chocolate, cakes and biscuits. She also gave me a magnesium supplement. After about three days, my symptoms started to improve. I had more energy and my periods became much less painful.

Adenomyosis

Tissue that is normally lining the womb can get into the muscular wall of the womb, where it sometimes forms nodules that may be confused with fibroids (see Chapter 3). The condition often goes undiagnosed. If you've got terrible period pain but there are few signs of endometriosis in the pelvic cavity, it's important to ask your doctor if you could have adenomyosis.

A vaginal ultrasound scan (see Chapter 3, the section on fibroids) can give a fairly accurate picture of what's happening inside the muscle and distinguish between fibroids and adenomyosis. Unlike fibroids, adenomyosis deposits can't be removed. An MRI scan is even better at helping to diagnose the condition, but even so cannot be 100 per cent accurate. Sadly, the only way to be completely certain is to check the womb muscle for deposits after a hysterectomy.

The treatments for adenomyosis are the same as for endometriosis. Thus, the combined pill can be taken to stop your cycles for several months, but not everyone can or wants to take the Pill. Also the Mirena IUS, which thins the lining of the womb and so reduces the actions of the deposits in the womb muscle, may prove helpful, but this, too, is a contraceptive and so is not suitable for those wanting to have a baby.

Key points

Don't put up with period pain. There are so many options, you should be able to find something to suit your circumstances. Conventional drugs, supplements and complementary therapies can provide pain relief and lifestyle changes can also make a big difference. See your doctor for advice on whether or not there is an underlying reason for the discomfort and what treatments would be best for you. Endometriosis is one of the chief suspects when it comes to severe period pain.

3
Heavy periods

Heavy periods are messy, difficult to deal with and can leave you feeling exhausted, but they're a fact of life for many women. They have to develop strategies each month to try and manage – wearing maximum protection, constantly having to change towels and tampons, carrying loads of sanitary protection round with them and making sure that they're never too far from a toilet. Some women have heavy periods throughout their childbearing years, while others may develop them at some point during this time. According to one set of figures, around 1 woman in 20 between the ages of 30 and 49 sees her GP each year with this problem. Of course, this statistic doesn't include women who just put up with the problem and manage on their own as best they can.

Hysterectomy (when the womb is removed surgically) has, until relatively recently, been the usual way that doctors have dealt with heavy periods. It's calculated that around 1 in 5 women has this operation before the age of 60, and 50 per cent of these women have the operation because of heavy periods. However, the womb is normal and not diseased in half of the women who have a hysterectomy for this reason.

The operation guarantees the end of periods and some women are very happy with the results, but it's a major operation and so carries certain risks. It's also not a solution for women who want to have children and some women want to keep their womb regardless of whether or not they plan to become pregnant. Luckily today hysterectomy is just one of a series of treatment options for women who suffer from heavy periods, so it's a case of weighing up the pros and cons of each treatment and what's right for you.

What is a heavy period?

It's really difficult to define this and it's hard to know whether or not your monthly blood loss is normal, particularly if you've always had heavy periods as this is all you know! Technically, heavy periods – or menorrhagia to give them their medical name – are described

33

as blood loss of more than 80 millilitres per period. Weighing menstrual loss is quite a business and not an exact science, though it's one way in which a decision can be made as to whether or not a woman is losing a lot of menstrual blood.

As noted earlier, women themselves find it hard to know what's normal. Some women who complain of heavy periods may lose less than 80 millilitres of blood, while others who have much heavier loss don't think that they have a problem. However, if the following sorts of things are happening to you, you're likely to have a problem:

- if you have to double up protection (use tampons and towels together) or use loads of tampons and pads (more than nine pads or tampons a day, according to some advice)
- if you pass clots, which are lumps that look a bit like liver
- having 'accidents', when you've stained your clothes or furniture
- flooding, where the blood gushes out
- worrying about where the nearest toilet is when you leave home or not going out for fear of having an 'accident'.

If you are passing clots, the reason for this is that, when there's bleeding, the body works to stop the blood loss by trying to achieve a balance between blood clotting and not clotting too much. Haemostasis is the term used for the process by which the body stops bleeding and various mechanisms are involved in this. Under normal circumstances, there are substances called fibrinolytics in the womb that make sure blood doesn't clot too much. If you're bleeding heavily, though, there aren't enough of these substances and the result is clots. Often what happens is that you get pooling of blood in the upper vagina and clots form there during the night, which then come out together with blood when you get up in the morning.

Heavy bleeding can lead to exhaustion and have a drastic effect on women's lives. A survey by the charity Women's Health asked women how they coped with heavy periods and found that, among other things, some had coped with heavy periods for a relatively short time of six to eight months, while others had lived with the problem for several years – some for as long as 20 years. Women reported having to get up in the night to change sanitary wear and soiled bedclothes. Some women were effectively housebound, using incontinence pads and plastic pants in addition to sanitary protection to cope. The heavy bleeding dominated their lives and they worried constantly about the problem.

The causes of heavy periods

There's a long list of reasons for periods becoming heavy, but often there isn't a clear-cut explanation.

Dysfunctional uterine bleeding (DUB)

This is a common diagnosis and simply means that there's no obvious reason for the problem. DUB is also used as a shorthand term for excessive or prolonged or frequent bleeding when there's no obvious disease. According to one estimate, DUB affects around 30 per cent of women at some point – most commonly women in their thirties and forties, when between 5 and 10 per cent may suffer from the problem.

DUB may occur if the delicate balance of hormones that govern the monthly cycle is out of kilter – the womb is fine, it's just that the messages it gets are disordered. This may happen in anovulatory (eggless) cycles when there's an imbalance of hormones because ovulation hasn't taken place so there's not enough progesterone in the second half of the cycle. Young girls who have started to have periods and women who are approaching the menopause are particularly likely to have these often irregular cycles that result in very heavy bleeding. However, this sort of bleeding can also happen in ovulatory cycles and is probably also due to disordered hormones.

Stress is definitely implicated in some cases of DUB and infections may also play a part.

Miscarriage

This can cause heavy bleeding – see the note on this under the heading Stopping prolonged bleeding and getting cycles back again, later on in this chapter.

Iron deficiency anaemia

Being deficient in iron can make periods worse. It is a vicious cycle, though, as women with heavy periods are at risk of developing this form of anaemia precisely because of their heavy blood loss each month. To make matters worse, once you're anaemic, your periods may get even heavier, though it's not clear why this happens.

35

Age

As you get older, you're more likely to have heavy periods, as we saw in the section on DUB above. It has been estimated that around 1 in 4 women aged 41–49 has heavy periods, 1 in 7 between 31 and 35 and less than 1 in 20 aged 19–25.

Fibroids

These are non-cancerous growths in the womb wall and are one of the commonest causes of heavy periods. They can cause severe bleeding. For more on fibroids, see the section describing the different kinds and options for treatment near the end of this chapter.

Diseases

Various diseases can cause heavy periods as a side-effect. For instance, liver disease may change hormone levels and make periods heavier. Heavy periods are also a common side-effect of kidney disease.

Polyps

These are non-cancerous lumps in the neck of the womb – the cervix – and can cause problems.

Endometriosis

You will recall that we discussed endometriosis in the last chapter. It can make periods not only more painful but also heavier.

Adenomyosis

This problem was also mentioned in the last chapter. It can make periods heavier as well as more painful.

Underactive thyroid gland

This can result in heavy bleeding during a period.

IUDs

These can make periods heavier and more painful. If your periods are already heavy, ask if it's a good idea to have an IUD fitted. If your periods have become heavier since having one inserted, you may want the IUD removed. Your decision will depends on the scale of the problem and whether or not you feel pain too.

Sterilization

Some women find that their periods are heavier after they have been sterilized. As discussed in Chapter 1, doctors say that there's no reason for this to be the case and that it may be due to the fact that women are getting used to their own natural cycles again after having been on contraceptives such as the Pill before being sterilized.

Sue, who was sterilized when she was 38, isn't convinced. She says that her periods got much heavier afterwards and that she had natural cycles before the operation as she wasn't using a hormonal contraceptive. If you're thinking about being sterilized, it's a good idea to ask your doctor about whether or not your periods could be affected. The risk of problems developing should be lessened as techniques have improved in recent years. One of the latest ones – 'Essure' – involves no cutting and has been likened to having an IUD fitted.

Smokers

Those who smoke have an increased risk of suffering from a range of period problems, including heavy bleeding.

Oestrogen dominance

As we have seen, hormonal imbalances can occur not only in eggless cycles but also in women who're overweight, as they make more oestrogen. The result may be heavier periods.

Bleeding or clotting disorders

Such disorders can cause heavy periods. For instance, women who carry the haemophilia gene can find that they have heavier periods than other women.

Von Willebrand's disease This is one of the commonest bleeding disorders. It's usually inherited and normally described as rare, but may affect as many as 1 in 100 women, according to some studies.

Von Willebrand's factor is a sort of glue that works by allowing blood cells, known as 'platelets', to stick on to damaged blood vessels to stop the blood flowing out. In type 1 von Willebrand's disease, which is the commonest form, there's a shortage of the factor so bleeding takes longer to stop. In type 2, the factor doesn't work properly and, in type 3, no factor is usually produced.

Symptoms of the disorder include heavy periods as well as frequent nose bleeds, skin that bruises easily and abnormal bleeding after surgery and childbirth.

Rona, 40, has type 1 von Willebrand's disease.

I've always had heavy periods. They used to last for about a week and were really bad for the first five days. I suffered from clots and flooding and used to have to wear towels and tampons together – I was always worrying about leaking and had to make sure I was near a toilet.

My brother has severe haemophilia and, in my early twenties, I was tested to see if I was a haemophilia carrier. That's when they discovered that I had von Willebrand's. I've tried various treatments and in 1997 took part in a trial of a nasal spray of a drug called desmopressin. It worked and I've been on it ever since and the good thing about it is that I need only use it for the first couple of days of my period.

There are several treatment options for heavy periods for women who have von Willebrand's disease, such as the treatments discussed below and desmopressin, as in Rona's case. Extra amounts of clotting factor VIII may be needed for women who have the type 3 form of the disease. If you suffer from heavy periods, they 'run in the family' and you also have the other symptoms described, it's worth finding out more about von Willebrand's disease. The Haemophilia Society produces a helpful booklet on the condition (see Chapter 10 under Bleeding disorders for contact details).

Getting help and a diagnosis

It's worth seeing your doctor to find out what can be done if heavy bleeding is interfering with your everyday life. You may be reluctant to go because you fear invasive tests and treatments, but initial diagnostic tests are usually not invasive. Talking the problems over with your doctor is often a very reassuring process, too, and you get a chance to find out about treatment options. Having said that, some women will decide to cope on their own. Louise suffered from very heavy periods, got medical help for the times when she bled excessively, but decided to keep going on this basis because she knew she was near the menopause.

The Royal College of Obstetricians and Gynaecologists has guidelines for doctors on how they should investigate and treat heavy periods when a woman first visits her GP and what sort of help she should receive if she has to be referred to a hospital. It is worthwhile taking a look at these so that you are informed and to ensure that you receive the best help. Key recommendations regarding what the best treatments are can be found in the next section.

As mentioned, the initial tests and checks that your doctor will do should be relatively simple and straightforward. Your GP will want to know what your periods have been like and will probably do a pelvic examination. It's also important that you should be tested for iron-deficiency anaemia. Iron is an essential part of haemoglobin, which is the oxygen-carrying pigment component in the blood. Iron deficiency reduces haemoglobin levels. Signs and symptoms may include:

- pale lips, tongue and nailbeds or the inside of the lower eyelids
- feeling weak
- dizziness
- breathlessness, particularly after exercise
- sometimes a fast heartbeat.

The only way to know for sure whether or not you are anaemic is to have a blood test. This should measure haemoglobin levels but also iron (ferritin) stores in the body, as these are depleted before haemoglobin levels start to go down.

Plenty of iron-rich foods, such as liver, meat, whole grains, fish and green leafy vegetables, can help, but, as Ann found, in the first instance, you'll need to take iron tablets to build up iron stores again.

My periods were heavy – that was a fact of life with which I coped – but they got heavier after my father died. Climbing stairs became a real effort and I remember my legs felt leaden. I never thought about it until a nurse I knew mentioned that she didn't think I looked very well and might be anaemic. So I visited the doctor's and had a blood test done. The surgery rang me a few days later to say I was severely anaemic. I was prescribed iron tablets for several months, started to feel better and blood tests showed I was no longer anaemic.

A thyroid test won't usually be done at this stage unless you have other signs that suggest an underactive thyroid, such as unexplained weight gain, hair loss, croaky voice, feeling depressed and sluggish.

More investigations may be needed if initial treatments aren't successful in order to try and find out the reason behind the heavy bleeding. These may include an abdominal scan, a transvaginal ultrasound scan (where a small probe is inserted into the vagina) or viewing the inside of the womb with an instrument called a hysteroscope. Sometimes a biopsy (a tiny sample of the womb lining) may be taken for analysis.

If you've got unusual bleeding, such as spotting after sex or bleeding in between periods (see Chapter 5), you may need these more detailed investigations at an earlier stage. It's very unlikely, but it's important to rule out rare but potentially serious conditions such as cancer of the womb or cervix.

Treatments

These divide mainly into drugs and surgical options, but there are some natural therapies and so on that may be worth a try. What is most appropriate for you will depend not only on the advantages and disadvantages of each treatment, but also on whether or not you want to have treatments that affect your fertility.

GPs should be able to help in the early stages and it's best to try and see a doctor in your practice who has a special interest in heavy periods. You may need to be referred to a gynaecologist if your problems are more complicated or if your GP seems uninterested in the problem.

Specialists should know about the latest treatment approaches and best ways to use the treatments available to help you. They may experiment with different approaches – for instance, perhaps prescribing a drug for longer than the normal guidelines state – but they should explain this and the potential risks involved so that you can make an informed choice about whether or not you want to follow this or another course of treatment.

Drugs

Tablet treatments can work really well, but you need to give the drug a chance to see if it works. It's recommended that you try it for three months and, if it hasn't worked by then, ask about other options. However, obviously don't wait that long if the bleeding is getting worse or the drug is giving you unpleasant side-effects.

It's important to realize that it is possible to find a drug works well for you even if the research suggests it's not the most effective treatment, so it's important to keep an open mind. For instance, tranexamic acid (discussed next) would normally be the drug of first choice for heavy periods, but you may find that, in your case, mefenamic acid suits you better. The point is that there is a choice, so, if one doesn't work very well, ask to try the other.

Tranexamic acid (Cyklokapron)

This is the best drug for heavy periods and is available on prescription. The only problem is that doctors don't usually offer it to women! One study found that only 5 per cent of GPs prescribed it, yet research shows that it can reduce bleeding by 50 per cent and it doesn't affect fertility, so can be taken if you want to become pregnant at some point. It's also only taken for around four to six days a month, just before and during your period.

It's an antifibrinolytic drug, which means that it inhibits fibrinolysis – the process in which fibrin, the main component in blood clots, is broken down. What this means is that, in order to reduce bleeding, the drug slows down the body's natural process of breaking down a clot.

Tranexamic acid works best if it's taken a day or two before your period is due until the bleeding has eased. This can be a problem if you don't know when your period is due, but, if you can tell when you ovulate (some women get twinges and a bit of pain and cervical mucus, which is a bit like egg white, increases), then count 14 days from then to calculate when it is due to start. You will usually be advised to take a 1-g tablet three times a day for up to four days.

As with any drug, it can have side-effects and these can include headaches, dizziness and nausea. There's no evidence that it can cause clots, but, if you've had clots in the past, it may not be an appropriate treatment for you.

Mefenamic acid (Ponstan)

This is the next best prescription treatment and is a non-steroidal anti-inflammatory drug (NSAID).

Mefenamic acid was first discussed in the last chapter as it reduces prostaglandin production and so helps relieve period pain. It also reduces bleeding by around 30 per cent and is very popular with doctors, so it may be the first drug that your doctor suggests. If you've got pain as well as heavy bleeding, therefore, it may be the best first choice, but, if not, ask about trying tranexamic acid first.

Mefenamic acid is best taken a day or so before your period starts. The standard dose is 500mg three times daily, which it is wise to take after meals on a full stomach as it may irritate an empty one.

Depending on the symptoms and severity of blood loss, you could also ask if it's worth taking tranexamic acid and mefenamic acid together, so that you get both pain relief and the maximum reduction in blood loss (50 per cent). However, you're unlikely to get more than a 50 per cent reduction in blood loss by combining the two drugs. One research study found that you get a 50 per cent reduction, not an 80 per cent (50 from tranexamic acid, plus 30 from mefenamic acid) reduction.

Vitamin E supplement

This option may be worth considering. Vitamin E, as noted in the last chapter, has been found to reduce pain and bleeding. It may be worth trying it in addition to the prescription treatments, but double-check that it's safe to do so.

Combined pill

This is very good for treating heavy periods because it does away with the monthly cycle and natural periods so that you just get a light withdrawal bleed. Taking the Pill each day, you will recall, means that you have relatively high levels of oestrogen in the body, as a result of which the pituitary gland stops producing follicle-stimulating hormone (FSH), so ovulation doesn't happen.

In the monophasic pill, the combination of constant doses of the two hormones oestrogen and progestogen, taken for 21 days, keeps the womb lining very thin. The result is that the withdrawal bleed is very light in the seven-day Pill-free break.

As mentioned in Chapter 2, the Pill isn't suitable for all women. Some find that it disagrees with them and some don't want to take it. There are, however, many different preparations, so if you want to take it but one doesn't suit you, ask about others.

Mirena IUS

This treatment became available in the UK about ten years ago. You will recall from earlier in the book that it's a contraceptive. It is a plastic IUD that releases levonorgestrel – a type of progestogen – directly into the womb. To recap, the Mirena works in several ways to prevent a pregnancy. It keeps the womb lining so thin that an embryo can't implant in it, thickens cervical mucus so that sperm can't pass through it and suppresses ovulation in some women, though most still ovulate while using the Mirena. An advantage is that oestrogen is still produced, so bone health is protected.

The Mirena works very well as a contraceptive, but was found to be so good at reducing heavy periods that it's now also licensed as a treatment for heavy periods. It results in a 90 per cent reduction in blood loss and 1 in 5 women will stop having periods within a year. The Mirena can be left in place for up to five years and, once it's removed, fertility returns. It has far fewer side-effects than taking progestogen as a tablet treatment, because the progestogen acts locally in the womb, so a much lower dose of it is needed.

Research in hospitals has shown that women can avoid having a hysterectomy if they have a Mirena. A large study, the Eclipse trial, is investigating the cost and effectiveness of the Mirena compared to standard treatments such as tranexamic acid, mefenamic acid and the combined pill in a GP setting.

The disadvantages of the Mirena are that most women will have irregular bleeding for the first three months or so, but this should settle down by around six months. There may also be temporary side-effects, such as headaches and breast tenderness, the IUS can sometimes be expelled and there's a slight risk of perforation when it's inserted. It's also not suitable for everyone. For instance, if you have pelvic inflammatory disease or a sexually transmitted infection, the insertion of the Mirena could allow the infection to get into the pelvis. Also, the womb has to be a certain length for the Mirena to be successfully inserted, but most women can have it fitted.

The Mirena is a little bit wider than a copper IUD so may be a bit more uncomfortable to fit for women who haven't given birth vaginally. This shouldn't normally be a problem, however, because a local anaesthetic can be given when the Mirena is fitted. Insertion usually takes between 5 and 15 minutes and should be done by a doctor experienced in fitting them. Afterwards, you may have a few cramps for several hours, but they should then stop.

Gonadotrophin-releasing hormone (GnRH) analogues

If the above hormonal treatments don't work or aren't an option for whatever reason, more powerful drugs like these and the others described below can be used. However, they're not the treatment of first choice because of their side-effects. Nevertheless, they may give you some time to consider your options or tide some women over until the menopause.

Sometimes also called gonadorelin analogues, examples are buserelin and goserelin and they can be administered in various ways – nasally or by injection, for example. They have the effect of overstimulating the whole hormonal system so that it shuts down. This creates a temporary menopause, which is good news if you've been suffering from heavy bleeding. However, the downside is that, because of the lack of oestrogen in your body, you're likely to experience the other less welcome menopausal symptoms, such as hot flushes, night sweats and vaginal dryness. Bone thickness can also be affected the longer you are on these drugs, so the normal advice is to take them for no longer than six months, though some specialists may prescribe them for longer if they think it's in your best interests.

Doctors usually give what's called 'addback therapy', which is HRT (an oestrogen and progestogen supplement), together with the GnRH, in the lowest possible dose to minimize the side-effects of the GnRH drugs. There are all sorts of HRT preparations, so ask about which is best and safest for you to take and for how long. The Committee on Safety of Medicines has issued guidance about the safe use of HRT and, essentially, it advised that it should be used for the shortest possible time and in the lowest dose for the relief of menopausal symptoms. (See Chapter 10 for details of where to find out more about official advice on the safety of drugs.)

Danazol

This is a drug that has anti-oestrogenic and anti-progestogenic effects in the body. It inhibits the release of the hormones produced by the pituitary gland and also suppresses the full development of the lining of the womb.

A dose greater than 400 mg a day usually results in periods stopping – amenorrhoea, mentioned earlier – in the majority of women. A 200-mg daily dose, though, will usually result in lighter periods and may also reduce period pain.

Despite these benefits, Danazol has major drawbacks as its masculinizing action can cause a long list of unpleasant side-effects, such as weight gain, acne, facial hair, disrupted sleep and fluid retention. As a result, it's just used as a short-term treatment – normally for three months.

Stopping prolonged bleeding and getting cycles back again

Progestogen When we're talking about heavy period treatments, it's a good idea also to mention the problem of prolonged bleeding.

Progestogen treatment can be used to stop prolonged bleeding and to re-establish cycles, but not to treat heavy periods (see the section below, What doesn't work for heavy periods?). It would be prescribed, for instance, if you haven't had a period for some weeks, then bleeding starts and won't stop.

Miscarriage is one of the commonest reasons for prolonged bleeding in women in their twenties and thirties, so it's important to see your doctor to rule out this possibility. Otherwise, this sort of bleeding may occur in women coming up to the menopause or in teenagers starting to have periods.

Treatment consists of progestogen tablets (usually a type of progestogen called norethisterone) taken for ten days. This will stop the bleeding. Once you have finished the tablets, you'll have another period. Then, on day 15, you'll take progestogen tablets again for 12 days. Again, once this course is finished you'll have a period.

Cyclical taking of progestogen like this will normally be prescribed for about three cycles to help your own cycle establish itself.

What doesn't work for heavy periods?

There are a couple of treatments that won't reduce blood loss, according to the Royal College of Obstetricians and Gynaecologists.

Low-dose norethisterone treatment This is still commonly prescribed in the second part of the cycle in the form of drugs such as Primolut N, when 5 mg will be taken twice daily from days 19–26 of the cycle to reduce bleeding. There's no evidence that it does this, though, and, ironically, if it is prescribed this way it may in fact increase bleeding.

Taking a higher dose of progestogen throughout the cycle can reduce heavy periods, but, as we saw above, has unpleasant side-effects, such as bloating and breast tenderness. Also, taking high doses of progestogen in the long term may damage blood vessel walls.

Ethamsylate This is the same sort of drug as tranexamic acid, but the evidence points to it not being anywhere near as effective.

Surgical options

There are other options if drugs don't work.

Endometrial ablation techniques (thinning the womb lining)

These techniques first became available about 20 years ago and were developed as an alternative to hysterectomy so that women had a less invasive treatment option.

What are known as first-generation techniques (the older ones), include transcervical resection of the endometrium (TCRE). This is a procedure in which the lining of the womb is removed with a wire loop, roller ball or laser. The choice of instrument depends on the surgeon's preference. The operation is performed using a hystero-scope, which is an instrument like a telescope. It is inserted through the vagina into the womb so that the surgeon can see inside. The lining is then destroyed.

Endometrial ablation should result in much lighter periods and some women stop having them altogether, but problems can recur and some may need to repeat the surgery. This treatment is not recommended if you want to have children as an embryo may not be able to implant properly in the womb lining after it has been treated.

In comparison to hysterectomy, these techniques have been seen as less risky, with a quicker recovery time, though there is still some risk of the womb wall being cut or of damage to the bowel and bladder.

An alternative to these techniques are the newest endometrial ablation techniques. In 2004, the National Institute for Clinical

Excellence (NICE) – the NHS medical watchdog – recommended two more recent techniques as treatments for heavy periods. However, NICE also noted that the older techniques should remain available because they may be the most appropriate option for some women. The newest techniques can usually be done under local anaesthetic, which makes them convenient.

First, there are the fluid-filled thermal balloon endometrial ablation (TBEA) devices, such as Cavaterm and Thermachoice. With such devices, a deflated balloon is gently inserted into the womb through the vagina and cervix. The balloon is then filled with heated liquid to destroy the womb lining, which comes away during the next few days.

Results show that bleeding returns to normal or is much lighter in around 85 per cent of women who receive this treatment. However, TBEA may not be suitable for women who have large, irregularly shaped wombs. Also, if you're allergic to latex, it's important to check that the balloon used is made of silicone.

The second technique is to use microwave endometrial ablation (MEA) – the Microsulis MEA system. This involves a probe being placed in the womb via the vagina and then using it to send out microwaves that destroy the lining of the womb.

Some studies report it as being at least as effective as TBEA and may be even more so. MEA may also be suitable for women who have an irregularly shaped womb cavity. This can occur as a result of having fibroids, though whether or not the technique can be used in such cases depends on the size and position of these growths.

It is recommended that an injection of a gonadotrophin-releasing analogue, such as buserelin, is given to help thin the lining of the womb a month before surgery is performed. If you have this done, you may experience temporary menopausal symptoms, which could last for around four to eight weeks.

As with the older techniques, there are possible complications, such as infections and perforation of the womb wall. You may also not be a suitable candidate if, for instance, you've had a certain type of incision in the abdominal wall, such as for a Caesarean, or if you've had other surgery on the womb that has left a scar on the womb wall so that it is less than 8 mm thick.

The newer techniques are said to be less dependent on the skills of the surgeon for their success than the earlier methods. The surgeon does not have to view the womb lining, as is required to perform the older techniques, but, obviously, problems may occur if the equipment is faulty. *Preserving Your Womb*, by Peter O'Donovan with Josephine Waters (Bladon Medical Publishing, 2004), has a helpful overview of the various endometrial ablation techniques.

Hysterectomy

Many women are very happy with this operation. It provides a permanent solution to the problems of heavy periods. If you're interested in this option, it's a good idea to discuss which type of hysterectomy is best for you.

The options include a total abdominal hysterectomy, in which the womb and cervix are removed through the abdomen. One or both ovaries can also be taken out in this operation, in which case it's called a total hysterectomy with bilateral (both ovaries removed) or unilateral (one removed) salpingo-oophorectomy. This is most likely to be advised if one or both ovaries are diseased, but some doctors are keen on removing healthy ovaries so that there's no chance of ovarian cancer developing at a later date.

If both ovaries are removed, you'll go into an immediate · menopause and may have severe menopausal side-effects due to the sudden stopping of oestrogen production. A paper presented by researchers at the Mayo Clinic in the USA, on 13 April 2005, to the American Academy of Neurology in Miami, has linked removal of both ovaries to an increased risk of developing Parkinson's disease – possibly because oestrogen production stops. It's important to check if the ovaries really do need to be removed and, if so, what options you have when it comes to HRT. As I mentioned in the section on GnRH drugs above, however, there are some safety concerns about HRT.

A sub-total hysterectomy, in which just the womb is removed, is a smaller operation and there's less risk of damage to the bladder occurring with it. The cervix is left in place, which is another consideration as some women report feeling less sexual satisfaction after it's removed. Some doctors are reluctant to leave the cervix in place in case cervical cancer develops at some point, but, if you've always had normal smears, this shouldn't be a problem, provided you keep on having smears done.

In a vaginal hysterectomy, the womb and cervix are removed through the vagina. This option may not be possible, however, if your womb is very large.

48

A hysterectomy is a major operation and recovery usually takes several months. Potential complications include bladder and bowel damage, wound infection and there's also a tiny risk of death – about 1 per 1000.

Some women may also have an earlier menopause than they would otherwise have done, even if the ovaries are not removed, if the blood supply to them is affected by the operation.

Natural therapies

The Mooncup

Sanitary protection is obviously a very important issue if you have heavy periods. A menstrual cup called the Mooncup could be worth considering. It's claimed that the Mooncup (a washable, reusable silicone cup) holds more fluid than a typical tampon or towel – three times as much, in fact – so it doesn't need changing so often (every four to eight hours) and leaks are less likely with it. There are two sizes depending on your age and whether or not you've given birth. (See Chapter 10 for sources of information about the Mooncup and suppliers.)

Diet and exercise

Watching what you eat and taking more exercise can help to rectify the hormonal imbalance that can wreak havoc with periods. Too much oestrogen and too little progesterone makes for heavy bleeding. If you're overweight, you may be more prone to heavy periods because fat produces more oestrogen than lean tissue.

Severe and chronic stress can also make periods heavy. Watch out for the effects on your period if, for instance, you're working very hard, exhausted by family commitments, have exams or have recently suffered a bereavement.

Eating a varied diet with plenty of fruit and vegetables will help. Also, make sure that you choose ones that are of various colours – red tomatoes, green leafy vegetables and different coloured peppers, for example – as these will give you lots of antioxidants, which help with heavy periods. Also, such a diet will give you plenty of B vitamins, which are good for stress.

Make sure that you include iron-rich foods in your diet if you're prone to anaemia. Good sources are lean red meat, nuts, lentils, soya beans, sardines, dried apricots and whole grains. Avoid drinking tea, especially with meals, as the tannin in it can reduce iron absorption.

49

Keeping active, while reducing body fat, has the added advantage of being a great stressbuster. See Chapter 7 for more on stress control.

Herbs

Taking herbs can help, but it's best to see a qualified herbalist rather than simply self-treat. Plants that may be suggested include agnus castus, which can help to rebalance hormones, and shepherd's purse, which is used specifically for heavy bleeding.

Smoking

This can be a cause of heavy periods, according to research, so try to stop.

Fibroids

These growths are an important cause of heavy periods. In the past, women with troublesome fibroids were given no choice other than to have a hysterectomy, but now there are other options on offer.

What are fibroids?

They're non-cancerous growths that develop in various parts of the muscular womb wall.

The main types are:

- submucous fibroids, which grow from under the lining of the womb
- intramural fibroids, which grow in the middle of the wall
- subserous fibroids, which grow near the outer part of the womb wall and can bulge into the pelvic cavity.

Some women have just one fibroid but you may have several and they can vary in size from as small as a seedling through to the size of a large grapefruit or even larger.

Fibroids are very common, often cause no problems and usually develop in the twenties and thirties, though Afro-Caribbean women may get them in their teens. It's still unclear why they develop, though it's accepted that oestrogen makes fibroids grow, which explains why they usually shrink after the menopause as oestrogen levels fall.

One of the main problems they cause is heavy and sometimes painful periods. Large fibroids can make some women look pregnant (see Jane's story below). The growths are often picked up on routine abdominal examinations, but the best way to detect them is by having an abdominal ultrasound scan or, better still, a vaginal ultrasound, as the scanner can get closer to the fibroids and so give more detailed information about the growths. The procedure is painless, no sedative is needed and you don't need to have a full bladder, which you do with an abdominal scan. A tiny probe is simply put into your vagina and the only time it may feel a bit uncomfortable is when the probe pushes against the top of the vagina.

Medical treatments for fibroids

If you have heavy periods, fibroids have been diagnosed and these are thought to be causing the problem (whether or not they will do so depends on their location), some of the options listed above may work. The drug treatments mentioned, the Mirena or endometrial ablation techniques may be used. Treatment choice, as always, will be dictated by whether or not you want to have children at some point.

If drugs don't work, fibroids can be removed or reduced in size by using various other techniques, some of which are listed below. Some gynaecologists use myolysis, which involves using lasers to reduce the size of the fibroid (for more details about this and other options see my book *Coping with Fibroids*, Sheldon Press, 1997).

Myomectomy

This is the medical term for the surgical removal of fibroids. One way of dealing with fibroids is to cut them out, though fibroids can regrow. Removing fibroids shouldn't affect your fertility, though there can always be complications with surgery, as discussed below.

A myomectomy can be performed in various ways, depending on the size and position of the fibroids. The easiest way to remove small ones is by doing a hysteroscopic myomectomy. This involves the surgeon inserting a hysteroscope through the vagina into the womb and using special instruments with it to cut and remove the fibroids. It may be possible to do this under a light anaesthetic as a day case.

Larger fibroids may need to be removed by carrying out a bigger operation, known as a conventional myomectomy. The surgeon either makes an incision in the abdominal wall or, if possible, operates using keyhole techniques. In keyhole surgery, only tiny incisions are made in the abdomen, but the surgeon needs to be highly trained to do this and the operation may take longer.

Whichever technique is used, an abdominal myomectomy is a complicated operation that carries some risks and it's possible that it could turn into a hysterectomy if problems arise during the operation.

Focused ultrasound

This is a relatively new form of treatment that is still in the early stages of development as a means of dealing with troublesome fibroids (see Chapter 10 for details of where to find out more about this method).

Focused ultrasound is 5000 times more powerful than diagnostic ultrasound and can be used to destroy fibroids without having surgery. A magnetic resonance imaging (MRI) scanner is used to help focus the more powerful ultrasound waves on the fibroids.

This may be a treatment of choice for women who want to keep their childbearing options open, like Jane. Her periods used to be hassle-free – like clockwork, she said – but that all changed several years ago when she was 33.

I suddenly started flooding when I was on holiday in Greece, which I was totally unprepared for. After that, my periods became incredibly heavy. I got awful clots, needed to use maximum protection, but still worried about having an accident. For a couple of days each month I'd feel faint, nauseous and wiped out. Then my stomach started to get bigger and I felt a dragging sensation in my abdomen, so I decided to see my GP. He congratulated me and said, 'You're five months' pregnant'. When I explained I wasn't, he mentioned the word 'fibroids'. They were diagnosed after I had an ultrasound scan. I was advised to have a hysterectomy, but I refused point blank because I thought I might want another child at some point.

After doing some research I ended up having focused ultrasound as part of a research project. I lay inside an MRI scanner and ultrasound was targeted on to my stomach to treat the fibroids. I was partially sedated for the treatment, which was slightly uncomfortable, but it took only a couple of hours and I went home later that same day. I was really pleased with the treatment because my periods returned to normal for some months, but then they started to get worse again, though I understood the treatment could be repeated.

Uterine embolization

This is a treatment option that has been around for about ten years.

Tiny particles are injected into the womb's arteries, as a result of which the fibroids shrink and die because they are starved of blood. The technique is performed under local anaesthetic, but, because it can sometimes result in severe pain, women are usually kept in hospital for a day or two afterwards.

The results so far are encouraging, though it will only be clear in the future what the long-term effects are of the procedure. One centre that has carried out over 900 procedures, claims an 80 per cent success rate and some women have gone on to have successful pregnancies afterwards. As with any treatment there are risks – the two most serious ones being premature menopause and infection, which can sometimes mean that a hysterectomy becomes necessary. If you are considering it, it's important to have it done by a doctor who is an expert in the technique.

Jane decided to have uterine embolization when her periods started to get worse again after having had the focused ultrasound. After the uterine embolization procedure, her fibroids were substantially reduced in size – by around 75 per cent – and her periods returned to normal. She doesn't know if the fibroids will regrow, but the evidence so far is that they don't.

Ruth was 40 when she was diagnosed as having fibroids after suffering from very heavy periods.

I was told that I should have a hysterectomy, but I didn't want one, I couldn't accept that this was my only option and I didn't want to give up hope of having a child at some point. I also didn't want to take six weeks off work. I struggled on, coping as best I could, but I was flooding day and night and had to carry bags of towels and tampons round with me and was dashing to the loo all the time. I was exhausted because I wasn't sleeping properly and, on top of that, I was anaemic.

I decided to have uterine embolization. The operation was done on Monday, I was out of hospital by Wednesday and back at work the following Tuesday. I had some pain for a couple of days, but had been warned to expect this. The treatment was brilliant because my periods became normal and have stayed that way.

Natural treatments for fibroids

Diet

Dietary measures may help to control fibroid growth by reducing the amount of oestrogen in the body. Certainly reducing the amount of fat in your diet should reduce oestrogen levels substantially. Try to avoid big swings in blood glucose levels, too, as this can lead to more fat being laid down than when the levels are fairly even. Eat regularly, having four or five small meals daily, and have a small amount of protein – pulses, egg or cottage cheese, for example – and some complex carbohydrates – such as wholemeal bread – at each meal. Cut back on refined carbohydrates, such as alcohol and white bread. Plenty of fibre in the diet, too, should help to flush oestrogen out of the body.

Herbs

Herbs such as Beth Root, Lady's Mantle and American Cranesbill may reduce bleeding and fibroid size.

Homeopathy

Homeopathy may be worth trying, particularly early on before fibroids become large. In one trial, homeopathy was found to reduce abnormal bleeding and pain in a significant number of 84 patients. For the best results, remedies should be tailored to each woman.

Key points

There are lots of effective treatments on offer and lifestyle changes can make a significant difference, too. Key recommendations from the Royal College of Obstetricians and Gynaecologists about the best treatments are as follows:

- What works: tranexamic acid, mefenamic acid, the combined Pill, the Mirena, endometrial ablation, hysterectomy; and more powerful drugs such as danazol and GnRH analogues work, but shouldn't be used on a long-term basis because of their side-effects.

54

- What doesn't work: low-dose norethisterone given in the second part of the cycle (though it does reduce bleeding given in higher doses throughout the cycle, it can cause unpleasant side-effects) and ethamsylate (a non-hormonal drug in the dose usually recommended).

Here's a quick checklist of the medical and surgical treatments that should not affect fertility, but may to different degrees (check with your doctor): tranexamic acid and mefenamic acid, surgical removal of fibroids and uterine embolization. It's not clear yet whether this is the case for focused ultrasound.

Treatments that do affect fertility include the combined Pill, the Mirena, powerful hormonal drugs such as Danazol and GnRH analogues.

Treatments that end fertility are endometrial ablation techniques and hysterectomy.

4

Irregular or missed periods

What's irregular?

It sounds like common sense, but it's worth spelling it out. Women who have regular periods pretty much know when their next period will arrive and generally what to expect and prepare for in terms of the length of their period and the amount of bleeding they will have. Regular periods are a sign that you're ovulating, your hormones are reasonably in balance and that your cycle is in order.

Irregular periods mean that you're not ovulating all the time and there's some disorder in your cycle. They can be a nuisance and an inconvenience because you're never quite sure when you're going to have one and the length of the period and amount of bleeding may be unpredictable, too. The result is that you can't plan around your periods and you can't take medicines a day or two early to control pain and/or bleeding as discussed in Chapters 2 and 3 because you never know when you're going to have a period.

Periods are part of the menstrual cycle and gynaecologists refer to cycle length in order to define regular and irregular periods. For any particular woman's situation they can say whether or not the length of her cycle fits into an agreed range of what's considered regular or, if the cycles vary in length each time, whether or not that variation is regular or irregular. There are therefore two ways in which your cycle can be irregular.

As discussed in Chapter 1, the 'classic' regular cycle length is 28 days, but anything between 25 and 35 is still described as regular and some gynaecologists have an even broader definition of, say, 21 to 35 days or even 21 to 42 days. If your cycles don't fit into these ranges, you're likely to be told that you have irregular periods. The term used for infrequent periods – those that occur less frequently than every six weeks – is oligomenorrhoea.

You'll also be told that you have irregular periods if the length of your cycle varies by more than about two days each side of what's normal for you. So, if it keeps swinging – say, from 26 days to 42 days then 23 days, and so on – that would be thought of as irregular.

Another important point to mention again here is that the part of the cycle that varies in length is the first half of the cycle – the follicular phase. The luteal phase, which occurs after ovulation, is always around 14 days long. If you have very short cycles of, say, 18 days, you're very unlikely to be ovulating.

Missed periods

When periods stop for more than six months or more, the term amenorrhoea is used.

Missing the odd period or two is usually nothing to worry about. However, if you're trying for a baby and pregnancy tests keep being negative and you don't have any periods for six months, it's important to get medical advice in case there's an underlying reason for the amenorrhoea.

What can affect your periods?

Many things can upset the hormonal balance that is necessary for periods to be regular. The result can be menstrual chaos. Women do often go through times of menstrual disturbance and this can be quite normal, but it is usually a reflection of what's happening in other parts of their lives.

Stress

Stress is an important cause. If your periods have gone haywire or changed in some way, it's important to ask whether or not the reason for this could be stress. Stress can not only make periods heavier and more painful, acute stress can stop periods or make them less or more frequent. Family life, overwork, exams, bereavement – these are just some of the many things that can cause stress overload. Rachel's periods became more erratic in her first year at university, which she thinks had something to do with the pressure she was under at the time. Her periods became more regular after she started to swim and run on a regular basis, but have become less frequent again. She thinks that this is due to yet more stress at university.

Pregnancy

This is obviously one of the first things to check if your periods stop.

Too little fat

It's estimated that at least 22 per cent of a woman's body weight needs to be in the form of fat in order for women to ovulate. If it falls below 17 per cent, periods will stop. You're very unlikely to have a regular cycle if your body mass index (BMI – a calculation based on your weight (in kilograms) divided by your height squared (in metres)) is less than 18.5.

Being overweight

Carrying too much body fat can also cause problems by creating a hormone imbalance, as we saw earlier. Being overweight is therefore linked to irregular cycles.

See also the section on polycystic ovary syndrome (PCOS) below.

Breastfeeding mothers

If you are breastfeeding, you are unlikely to have regular cycles. They should return to normal once breastfeeding has stopped.

Ovarian cysts

These are growths on or inside one or both ovaries. There are various types and they may make periods irregular.

Over-exercising

Exercising frequently each week and intensive physical training can stop periods.

The time of the menarche

It's quite normal for teenagers to have erratic cycles when they start having periods – the menarche being the medical term for the onset of menstruation – as the hormonal system needs time to settle down.

Contraception

If you have been taking the Pill and then stop, this may result in you having irregular periods for a few months afterwards as it takes a little time for your hormonal system to re-establish itself.

Progestogen-only contraceptives – such as the progestogen-only pill – may cause irregular periods.

The menopause

The start of the menopause is often heralded by irregular periods several years beforehand. This is due to the hormonal fluctuations that occur at this time. You may have no periods for some months, then several very short cycles, then go back to having infrequent periods, with bleeding being light sometimes or very heavy. As Catherine discovered (Chapter 1), cycles can become very erratic.

If you've also started to get hot flushes – feeling uncomfortably hot for no obvious reason – this is another sign that you're perimenopausal, which means that you are approaching the menopause. Blood tests are sometimes done to measure FSH as rising levels may be an indication that you're perimenopausal. See also the section on ovarian reserve tests under the heading Do you need to have periods?, below. These tests can be used to assess how many eggs you have left if you are experiencing these kinds of symptoms and want to have children. The menopause (your last period) occurs when you have about 1000 follicles left.

Drugs

These can sometimes make periods stop or become irregular, so, if you're taking long-term medication and notice that your cycles have changed, there could be a link.

Medicines such as prednisolone – a steroid taken for its anti-inflammatory effect for various conditions, such as rheumatoid arthritis – may cause menstrual disturbance or make periods stop. Ask your doctor whether or not there are any other treatments on offer or if taking a lower dose of the drug might still be effective and mean that your periods return to normal.

Of course, hormonal contraceptives, such as the combined pill, stop your natural cycle and you have a withdrawal bleed instead.

Polycystic ovary syndrome (PCOS)

PCOS is an important cause of irregular or absent periods, so a more extensive section below is devoted to it.

Epilepsy

Women with epilepsy (around 200,000 women in the UK are affected) may find that they have irregular cycles. This may be due to the fact that seizures affect the release of the hormones that control ovulation.

Under- or overactive thyroid

The thyroid gland is an important hormonal gland in the body that regulates energy. An underactive or overactive one is an important cause of irregular or absent periods, as well as heavy periods.

Serious medical conditions

A serious problem, such as a tumour in the pituitary gland, may occasionally be the reason for the absence of periods.

Premature ovarian failure

By this is meant a premature menopause, which would be if it occurred before the age of 40.

It's often unclear why this happens, but it may run in families. Other reasons may include viral or bacterial infections, pelvic inflammatory disease, cancer treatments and smoking has been shown to lower the age of the onset of menopause.

Prolactin levels

Levels of this hormone can rise as a result of stress and cause periods to stop. Prolactin is a hormone produced by the pituitary gland that is responsible for the production of breastmilk.

Do you need to have periods?

Should you worry if you're having only the occasional period or none at all? There are several answers to this. Yes, if you want to become pregnant as regular periods are a sign that you're ovulating.

As we've seen, an approaching menopause is a perfectly natural reason for irregular periods. However, if you want to have a baby, ovarian reserve tests are now being offered by some fertility clinics as a way of trying to predict how many eggs are left so you can then work out what your options are. The tests aim to assess the number of eggs there are by measuring the volume of the ovaries, calculating the number of remaining egg follicles, measuring ovarian blood flow and sometimes levels of inhibin B, which is a hormone produced by the ovaries. Women with a family history of early menopause may find it helpful to have their ovaries assessed, but the tests are new and it's important to ask about their accuracy so you can make informed decisions.

If you don't want to have a baby, there are a couple of other points to consider. If you're not having periods, you may not be producing enough oestrogen, which your body needs to build strong bones in order to reduce the risk of developing the bone-thinning disease osteoporosis at a later date. However, lack of oestrogen isn't a problem for women with PCOS, even though they may have only infrequent periods or none at all.

Finally, having a regular bleed is a good thing as it gets rid of tissue that, if left where it is, may, in the longer term, increase the risk of developing cancer of the lining of the womb. This is a particular concern for women who have PCOS (see the section below).

Establishing a cycle

See your doctor to discuss whether or not you need to have tests to check if there's an underlying disorder, such as an over- or underactive thyroid, as this may be the reason for irregular or absent periods.

Lifestyle measures really can help hormones. Aim to achieve a balance between too little and too much. For instance, under-exercising or over-exercising can mess up your cycle, so have a look at what you're doing and see if any changes can be made (see Chapter 9 for more on exercise). Similarly, eating too little or too much can play havoc with your hormones (see Chapter 8 on diet).

Stress is a very important cause of menstrual disturbance, so, if you suspect that this is the reason for your irregular periods, look at ways in which you can destress your life. If, for example, you're working too hard, see if you can ease up and cut down on your work. Making various other changes can help, too. For instance, try to substitute positive for negative thoughts, ask for help if you need it, break tasks down into ones of a manageable size and make time to regularly enjoy practising relaxation techniques. Bear in mind, though, that you need to allow several months for lifestyle measures to have an effect on your cycle. (See also Chapter 7 on stress reduction.)

Medical treatments

If you've got an underlying disorder, such as an over- or underactive thyroid, you will need to have that treated first to see if it is responsible for the problem with your periods, only pursuing other treatments if the problem continues.

If you want to have a baby, fertility tests will need to be carried out and, depending on the results, you may need to take an anti-oestrogen drug called clomiphene to kick-start ovulation.

Otherwise, the following measures can help, but they will not treat an underlying cause of the problem.

- If you don't want to have a baby and are happy to take a hormonal contraceptive, the Pill can give you an artificial cycle with a regular withdrawal bleed.
- Progestogen, as we've seen, is used in various ways to stop or start bleeding (depending on the dose and how long it's taken for). Cyclical progestogen (see Chapter 3, the section on stopping prolonged bleeding), taken for three months, for example, may be suggested by some doctors to try and establish a normal cycle. After the three months, you would stop taking the progestogen and see if your cycle is normal. However, the tablet treatment can cause side-effects, such as bloating and breast tenderness. (See under the heading Shedding the womb lining, in the section on PCOS below if there are concerns that your lining is getting too thick.)

Polycystic ovary syndrome (PCOS)

This condition is an important cause of irregular or absent periods.

How PCOS affects women

It often develops at an early age and can have a drastic effect on women's lives.

Thirty-year-old Lucy remembers that she had her first period when she was 14. The bleeding didn't stop – it just went on and on. After two months, she was taken to see her doctor, who referred her for an ultrasound scan. The scan showed that her ovaries were covered in lots of cysts.

I saw a gynaecologist who put me on a type of Pill called Dianette and told me that if I wanted children I would have to have them very soon!

I stayed on the Pill till I was 16 and at that point started to develop hair on my face, like a man's beard, on my chin and sides of my face. I had electrolysis every week to remove the hair. Then, the tone of my voice started to drop and people thought I was a man when I was speaking to them on the phone.

I was still on Dianette, but my periods were getting heavier and I was also suffering from back pain and stomach cramps. My energy levels slumped. The withdrawal bleeds just wiped me out and I'd have to stay in bed for a couple of days to recover. So, I went back to the gynaecologist, who put me on various progestogens for six months, together with Dianette, to see if that would help.

The bleeding did improve, also the hair growth slowed down a bit and my voice became slightly higher again, which helped. Then I was put on a drug called Metformin together with the Dianette, but I felt wobbly on the Metformin. I lost less blood and needed less sanitary protection, but the blood was brown rather than red, my cramps became much worse, they didn't ease up and I felt really uncomfortable.

Apart from this, I've always had a weight problem from about the age of 18, when the weight started to pile on and became very difficult to shift – I'm probably about 5 stone overweight. The Metformin did help me lose a bit of it, but, after a few months, I couldn't take it any more because my periods were so painful.

I came off Dianette when my husband and I decided to try for a family, but I kept on bleeding, which was really scary, so I saw the gynaecologist again, who put me back on progestogen. I'm now on Yasmin – a different Pill that I've been on for about a couple of years. It's helped, but I'm starting to get a lot of breast pain now, so I don't know how much longer I'll be able to stay on it.

I do try to keep fit by going to the gym and I'm very careful about what I eat, but my periods exhaust me and I only feel human for about two weeks every month.

PCOS has had a huge effect on my life. I've become exhausted with the monthly bleeds and I'm chronically tired, which has affected my ability to work. I've shed a lot of tears about not being able to have kids because I do want children, but I'm scared of coming off the Pill, given what happened the last time round. There's another side to this, too. I wouldn't want to pass PCOS on to a daughter if I had one.

Susan was 34 when PCOS was diagnosed.

I started having periods at 15, then had one every few months, I

63

was put on the Pill between the ages of 17 and 20, but decided to come off it because I didn't like taking it and I wasn't sexually active. My periods became irregular again, though they weren't painful or heavy, and I put on weight.

I got married when I was 25 and was referred to a fertility clinic when I didn't get pregnant. They did various tests and told me to go away and only come back when I'd lost some weight, which I didn't manage to do.

My marriage broke up and I had no periods for a couple of years, so my mum thought I was going through the 'change'. I've got a new partner now and I've managed to lose some weight, which has dropped from 23 stone to 18 stone, so I'm attending the fertility clinic.

PCOS has been diagnosed and now I'm on Metformin all the time, but I think I'd be a lot slimmer if it wasn't for the PCOS. I go to Weight Watchers and swim at the pool at work whenever I can and managed to lose 5 stone, but it's been a real struggle. PCOS has really affected me a lot because I may never be able to have kids. I did conceive last year, but then miscarried.

What is PCOS?

This is a puzzling condition, which is called a syndrome because it is a collection of symptoms. Many women – as many as one in five – have polycystic ovaries, which means that they are covered in little cysts about 2 to 4 mm across. These form just underneath the outer surface of the ovaries and look like a string of beads on ultrasound scans.

Women who have polycystic ovaries usually ovulate normally as the ovaries are otherwise healthy. However, as many as 15 per cent of women (a figure that may well increase as the numbers of women who are overweight continue to rise – see the section headed Weight control and keeping fit, below) have not only polycystic ovaries but also suffer various problems. They have a mix of symptoms called polycystic ovary syndrome (PCOS), which can affect them in a number of ways.

In a normal cycle, about five egg follicles develop, but only one goes on to become dominant, growing to around 20 mm across. During this maturing process, the follicle makes oestrogen. The pituitary gland responds by releasing less FSH and LH, which means that the other follicles stop developing. What happens in PCOS, however, is that the ovaries have many more developing follicles and these start to grow, but then the process stops, so no dominant follicle emerges and ovulation does not usually occur.

Some of the symptoms can be distressing and embarrassing, but it's important to emphasize that the effects of this condition can be very variable. The most common symptom is irregular (infrequent) periods, which affects at least 60 per cent of women with PCOS (Lucy, Susan and Rachel, who tell their stories below, all have infrequent periods), followed by excess hair on various parts of the body, such as the face, chest, abdomen, arms and legs, the hair on the top of the head thinning, problems conceiving and, possibly, a higher miscarriage rate, being overweight and finding it difficult to lose weight, having no periods and acne. Many women with PCOS also have insulin resistance (see below, under the heading Hormones).

In the long term, women with PCOS may be more at risk of developing diabetes in mid life, heart disease and high blood pressure. Also, there is a danger of developing endometrial cancer, which is cancer of the lining of the womb, as the risks of this increase if the womb lining is not shed regularly. At one point, women with PCOS were thought to have an increased risk of developing breast cancer, but that's not thought to be the case now.

PCOS usually starts during adolescence, but may develop later on when women are in their twenties and thirties. Women who have this condition are affected by it in different ways – some having just a few of the symptoms, some having all of them, some only being affected mildly, while others have severe symptoms.

What causes PCOS?

Hormones

It's a complicated condition and the causes still aren't fully understood, but the main characteristic is hormonal imbalance and it's the most common hormonal disturbance to affect women.

Women with PCOS usually have abnormally high levels of LH, an androgen called testosterone, less FSH, more oestrogen and less progesterone. Testosterone is the most important of the male sex hormones produced by the ovaries as it needs to be there for oestrogen to be made, but in higher than normal amounts it leads to more body hair, acne and a deeper voice.

Too much insulin

Women may also have raised levels of the hormone insulin – produced by the pancreas. Insulin is vital for health as it regulates blood glucose, making sure that not too much of it builds up in the blood. The body needs to have stable amounts of this hormone in order to work properly.

With PCOS, some women develop what's called insulin resistance, which means that the body doesn't respond properly to insulin, so more insulin has to be produced. These higher insulin levels play some part in the picture of hormonal imbalance that is seen in PCOS. Higher levels of insulin may result in abnormal levels of cholesterol and fats, increasing the risk of developing heart disease and diabetes, and may stimulate the higher than normal testosterone levels in the ovaries.

Family link

There is a genetic element to the condition – that is, it develops due to faulty genes – so some women may inherit a tendency to develop PCOS. However, whether or not they actually do so depends on lifestyle factors. So, for example, women with polycystic ovaries may develop PCOS as a result of becoming overweight.

Epilepsy

Epilepsy is linked to PCOS – women with epilepsy have a higher risk of developing PCOS than the rest of the female population. They may also have an extra increased risk of developing it if they take the epileptic drug sodium valproate. Some doctors thus advise that women of childbearing age should be given alternative medication if at all possible. Women already taking sodium valproate should be screened for PCOS and, if they have it, be offered other medication. If you've just been diagnosed as having epilepsy, check what options you have.

Diagnosing PCOS

Various tests will be carried out if PCOS is suspected.

An ultrasound scan enables doctors to look at the ovaries. A vaginal ultrasound will give more detail than an abdominal scan and can show whether or not the ovaries have the tell-tale strings of cysts on their surface.

Various blood tests will be performed to rule out other conditions, such as abnormal thyroid function, and check various hormone levels. If you're having periods, the tests are usually carried out at the start of your cycle, as this gives a more accurate base level picture of what's happening to your hormones. If you're not having periods, the tests can usually be performed at any time but may need to be repeated depending on the results.

Treating PCOS

There's no drug that can be prescribed to cure the condition. Having said that, it can be successfully managed. Often, simply making adjustments to your lifestyle can have a positive impact and some doctors think that these steps may sometimes be sufficient in themselves to switch off the condition.

What steps you take will depend on what symptoms you have, their severity and whether or not you want to have a baby, as well as an assessment of what long-term health risks you may be prone to as a result of having PCOS.

Lifestyle and PCOS

Weight control and keeping fit

It's not true of all sufferers, but many women with PCOS are overweight, put on weight easily and yet find it difficult to lose it. What seems clear at the moment is that being overweight worsens PCOS symptoms such as excess hair, acne and infertility. The reason for this is that very overweight women produce more insulin and high insulin levels are likely to switch on the genes in the ovaries that increase testosterone levels and result in problems such as lack of ovulation, acne and excess body hair. Women with polycystic ovaries increase their chances of developing PCOS if they become overweight, but it can be very hard to lose weight, as Rachel explains.

Aged 24, Rachel was diagnosed as having PCOS when she was about 19 and has struggled with her weight ever since.

I started having erratic periods when I was 13 and, when I went to university, I didn't have one for six months, so I went for some

67

tests. PCOS was diagnosed after an ultrasound scan and various blood tests. I was put on the Pill to give me a cycle and regular bleeds. I also developed a bit of acne, and facial hair, which I have to pluck out regularly.

I've always been described as chunky, even though I used to be very active when I was at school and played games like hockey and did cross-country running. The weight has piled on as I've got older. I really do try hard to watch what I eat, but I've been on all sorts of diets that didn't work. It was only when I went on the Atkins and restricted my carbohydrate intake that the weight started to come off. I lost 2 stone, but it's been very hard to stick to the diet. I'm trying to get pregnant now and I still need to lose about 4 stone to get down to my ideal weight of 12 stone.

I'm on Metformin, 850 mg twice daily, which helps regulate my blood pressure and blood sugar. When I started on the drug I had dreadful wind and diarrhoea to start with, but I was warned about this and things have settled down.

My periods have been regular now for the last 11 months. At first they were around 32 to 34 days, but they're 28 days now. They're heavy and painful, but then they've always been like that so I put up with the discomfort. I was offered drugs to make my periods lighter, but I don't want to take anything else.

My husband and I have been together a year and it's hard to accept that I might never have kids as the rest of my family haven't had any problems having children. I keep fit and watch what I eat because I worry about my long-term health, but it's really hard to get my weight down. It's all been very difficult at times and I became depressed at one point and took antidepressants to help.

Finding out so young that I might have problems conceiving has been a burden because I wanted to travel round the world first before having children, but I don't want to get to a certain age and regret not having kids, so we've postponed the travel plans for now.

Many women with PCOS, like Rachel, find losing weight hard, but you don't have to lose a lot of weight for it to have a positive effect. Research shows that losing just 5–10 per cent of excess body weight can significantly improve symptoms. Rachel thinks that her periods became regular after she lost a couple of stone, though this may be in part to do with taking Metformin. As Rachel, Lucy and Susan say, losing weight hasn't been easy, but doctors agree that shedding weight and keeping it in check, even if you're not overweight, is important and a key first-line approach. It can reduce symptoms, may even switch off the disease and, in the long term, reduces the risk of developing diabetes.

One of the easiest ways to keep an eye on your weight to improve your short-term and long-term health is to check how much fat you're carrying round your middle. Aim for a waist measurement of not more than 81.5 cm (32 in) as, if it's over this, your risk of health problems starts to increase. A healthy body mass index (BMI) figure (see Chapter 8, under the heading Keep an eye on your weight) is ideally between 18.5 and 24.9.

When it comes to trying to improve the symptoms of PCOS, follow general healthy diet advice. See Chapter 8 on diet, but, in particular, choose to eat more of the carbohydrates that are digested slowly and release less insulin. This means foods with what's known as a low glycaemic index (GI). Doing this should help you to lose weight.

Carbohydrate foods that are quickly digested have the highest GI scores as they rapidly raise blood glucose levels and lead to a release of insulin to bring blood glucose back to a stable level. The GI value of various foods have been measured – low ones have a value of under 55, medium GI foods 56–69, high ones 70 and over. Aim to eat more of the low and medium GI foods and include the high ones sparingly. However, some high GI foods can be nutritious so, in order to benefit from them and not jeopardize your diet, eat them with low GI foods to reduce the high glucose response that the high GI foods will provoke. So, for example, you could have baked beans on toast as the beans have a low GI, but bread, depending on the type, has a higher GI.

The GI rating given to foods also depends on whether or not the carbohydrate has been mixed with other things, such as fat, and how much carbohydrate you're eating at a meal.

Low GI foods are thought to reduce hunger pangs because they're more slowly digested than other foods and that, of course, helps when you're trying to lose weight. Also, eat plenty of fibre as this slows the rate at which food is digested and make sure to go easy on sugary foods.

As a general rule, try not to skip breakfast – if you do, you may have hunger pangs later in the morning and succumb to something that has a high GI. Also, have regular meals and low GI snacks throughout the day, aiming to have most of your calories before 5 pm. The *PCOS Diet Book* by Colette Harris and Theresa Cheung (Thorsons, 2002) covers dietary advice in detail.

Keeping fit will help, too, even if you're overweight, as it makes your body better able to deal with blood sugar, which means you're less likely to develop insulin resistance. Aim to get slightly out of breath several times a week by, for instance, going for a brisk half-hour walk. Work out how to become more active in your everyday life – take the stairs rather than the escalator and so on.

Medical help for PCOS

Shedding the womb lining

Lack of oestrogen isn't a problem for women with PCOS, even though they may have only the occasional period. What is an issue, though, is whether or not the lining of the womb should be shed every so often to reduce the risk of developing endometrial cancer (cancer of the lining of the womb).

Current thinking is that something needs to be done to reduce this risk if you have fewer than three periods a year. However, some doctors think that, because the risk of this cancer is low in younger women, there's usually no need to do anything. They argue that it's only necessary to check the lining of the womb if you have abnormal bleeding. However, other doctors say that it's a good idea to induce a bleed about four times a year.

The easiest way to bring on a bleed is to take progestogen tablets, usually for about ten days, after which you'll have a bleed. However, progestogen can cause side-effects such as fluid retention, bloating and acne, which can be counter-productive. Another option, if you haven't had a bleed for a year, is for the thickness of the womb lining to be checked by doing a vaginal ultrasound and, if necessary, taking a biopsy, which is a tiny sample of the womb lining, and sending it for analysis.

Taking the Pill is another option as it gives you regular bleeds and it may also help with problems of acne and excess body hair. There are lots of different Pills, so it's a case of finding which one suits you as they vary in terms of their content and dosages of hormones. Yasmin contains an anti-androgen, which may be helpful for some

70

women suffering excess body hair and acne, as does Dianette, which is often prescribed for acne and excess hair. Against that you have to weigh up the fact that the Pill has side-effects, too, such as an increased risk of clots and it may increase insulin resistance. Finding the right one for you will depend on your family history, general health and mix of PCOS symptoms.

It is useful to know that some research suggests that cycles naturally become more regular as women with PCOS get older – that is, into their thirties and beyond. It may be a good idea, therefore, to stop the Pill every so often to see if this is happening. If it is, there's no need to stay on the Pill unless you want to use it for contraceptive purposes.

An alternative way of keeping the womb lining thin is to have the Mirena IUS fitted. You're likely to have some spotting and irregular bleeding for several months at first with this, but the erratic bleeding should stop. Most women go on to become period-free with the Mirena, which isn't a problem in this case as the Mirena keeps the womb lining very thin.

Acne and excess body hair

Yasmin and Dianette, as we saw above, can help with the masculinizing effects that some women experience. If you can't take the Pill, another option might be a drug called spironolactone. It's used to treat high blood pressure, but also has anti-androgen effects. The downside of this drug, however, is that it can cause irregular bleeding.

Vaniqa is a new prescription cream that works by slowing down hair growth so hair doesn't have to be removed as often. You need to allow a couple of months for it to start to work but if you've seen no benefits by four months it's unlikely to be effective for you.

Non-drug ways in which to remove excess hair include electrolysis and the old-fashioned methods of shaving, waxing and plucking it out.

Metformin

Metformin is a drug used to treat what's known as type 2 diabetes by helping to lower blood sugar. It's now also being used to help women with PCOS in a number of ways. It makes the body more sensitive to insulin, so reduces insulin resistance. It also lowers

71

testosterone levels, which reduces acne and excess hair and brings back regular periods and ovulation.

Metformin is taken continuously, rather than as a course, but can initially cause wind and gut problems, as Rachel discovered. For this reason it's usually taken in a lower dose for the first two weeks, then the dosage is increased to minimize these kinds of problems.

Other drugs that lower insulin resistance are rosiglitazone and pioglitazone, but much less is known about these drugs than Metformin. The advice is to avoid them unless you're taking part in a research trial, where you'll be carefully monitored.

Recent research suggests that the fat-blocking drug orlistat (Xenical) may help women with PCOS by helping to reduce excess weight and lowering testosterone levels, though more studies need to be done before it will become prescribed generally.

Becoming pregnant and PCOS

The first thing to do is lose weight in order to establish regular cycles and, with these, ovulation. If this doesn't happen, there are a number of other options.

Clomiphene

This is the usual drug of choice that is used to kick-start ovulation and it's usually taken on days two to six of your cycle. Clomiphene has an anti-oestrogen action. This means that it works by reducing oestrogen levels, which in turn makes the pituitary gland increase production of FSH, which means that there's a greater chance of one of the little follicles developing into a dominant one.

If it hasn't worked by six months, you'll normally be advised to try another treatment.

There are some other factors that you need to bear in mind with clomiphene. It is very good at causing women to ovulate, but can result in multiple births, so you need to think about whether or not you would be prepared to take this risk. Also, there are concerns from research carried out some time ago that clomiphene might increase the risk of ovarian cancer developing, though this hasn't been substantiated.

Drugs called aromatase inhibitors, used to treat breast cancer, also inhibit oestrogen and may become an alternative treatment to clomiphene in the next few years.

Metformin

This is probably the next drug of choice to encourage ovulation, though for some doctors it is their first choice. It's taken continuously, as described above, usually in doses of 1500 mg daily. However, some women find that they can't tolerate the side-effects associated with it, even when the dose is gradually increased over a period of time, which works for some women who have PCOS.

Other options

- Taking Metformin and clomiphene together can be tried to induce ovulation.
- Being given an injection of the hormone FSH for 12 to 14 days, followed by a hormone injection to trigger ovulation has a very high rate of success for resulting in pregnancy.
- Laser drilling works well, too – 75 per cent of women who don't ovulate will do so after about four tiny holes are drilled in to each ovary using a laser.

PCOS and long-term health

The right diet and regular exercise can help to reduce the risks of developing problems in the future.

Some women are keen to take Metformin on a long-term basis to reduce the risk of developing diabetes later on. At the moment, though, it's unclear if it can actually have this effect and whether or not there are any risks to taking it for long periods of time. As a result, doctors may be reluctant to prescribe it on this basis. You would probably need it to be prescribed for you by a specialist and then you should be carefully monitored thereafter.

Whether you are taking Metformin or not, it's a good idea to have annual checks anyway to pick up any early signs of diabetes. This is a doubly important precaution if you're overweight and have a family history of the disease.

Diabetes damages the body in various ways. As there's too much sugar in the blood, this may damage organs such as the eyes, heart, kidneys and nervous system, causing irreparable damage if it goes undetected or is not managed effectively.

A test for insulin resistance may be suggested to check your risk of developing diabetes. You need to have an empty stomach, after a night's fast, and a sample of blood is taken; then you have a sugar drink and a couple of hours later another sample of blood is taken. Tests are performed to measure the levels of insulin and glucose in each of the samples. If it is found that you are insulin resistant, then it's even more important to keep fit as well as lose weight to control the levels of glucose and avoid it causing damage to the body.

Complementary therapies for irregular/absent periods

These have a part to play, whether you choose aromatherapy, reflexology or other therapies, if they help you to relax, destress and give you a sense of control over your life.

Herbs such as agnus castus may be used for PCOS to help rebalance the hormones, but it's important to see a qualified herbalist rather than self-treat as your particular mix of symptoms and lifestyle factors could make this unsuitable for you. Which herbs are recommended will depend on the underlying cause of the lack of periods, but could include agnus castus, as mentioned, sage, liquorice or motherwort.

Key points

Don't panic if your periods go haywire – it's not unusual for this to happen at some point in every woman's life, particularly around the time of the menopause. The finely balanced hormones that govern the monthly cycle can also be disrupted by all sorts of factors, including stress and over-exercising. If pregnancy tests are negative and periods stop for more than six months or you're having infrequent periods, it's a good idea to see a doctor to find out what's going on.

5

Bleeding between periods

Bleeding between periods, after sex or after the menopause is known as irregular bleeding and is considered abnormal. This sort of irregular bleeding needs to be checked because occasionally it is a sign that something is seriously wrong. In particular, it can be a sign of cancer of the cervix or the womb and your doctor will be keen to exclude these possibilities.

Don't panic. Irregular bleeding is common and usually nothing is wrong. However, it is important to seek medical advice to find out, if possible, what's causing it. Apart from anything else, bleeding when you're not expecting it is annoying and, if it can be stopped, this makes life a bit easier!

What is irregular bleeding?

Odd bits of spotting, making light stains on underwear can be quite normal for some women who experience this, for instance, a couple of days before their period starts. Some women also have a light bleed or spot for a couple of days around the time that they ovulate. Keeping a diary and jotting down when this happens will show if there's a cyclical pattern to the bleeding, in which case no further investigations are likely to be needed.

In other situations, it can be difficult to know what's irregular bleeding as it isn't always obvious. If you have regular periods, it's usually easy to identify irregular bleeding because you know the shape and pattern of your periods – how bleeding starts, the sort of bleeding and how long it goes on for. If your periods are starting to become irregular or have always been irregular, though, then it can be harder to judge. Then, what might seem like irregular bleeding could, with hindsight, be just an irregular period.

It's easy to get confused in such cases. Catherine, for instance, thought that she had been through the menopause and had had her last period. A few months later, she started to bleed.

I was really frightened because I thought that this meant something was badly wrong. I panicked and didn't know what to make of the blood. So, I rushed off to see my GP, full of dread, but she was very relaxed about it and said she thought that it might be another period. She was right. It went on for three days and then stopped. It was at that point I realized, looking back at the pattern of the bleeding, that it was another period.

However, if you've just had a period and then started to bleed again a week later, that counts as irregular bleeding as it's too soon to have another period. If you're in any doubt, the best thing is to consult your doctor.

Why irregular bleeding occurs

Miscarriage

This is a common reason for unexpected, prolonged bleeding in women who are in their twenties and thirties.

It could also be a sign of an ectopic pregnancy. In this case, you'll experience one-sided abdominal pain as well as bleeding. If this happens, you need to seek medical treatment urgently.

Hormonal imbalance

This can easily occur as a result of factors such as stress. An imbalance in the hormones can upset the usual rhythm of your cycles and end up in abnormal bleeding. This is particularly likely if you're coming up to the menopause and not ovulating regularly. Your cycles may be all over the place and so it may be unclear whether you've got irregular bleeding or irregular periods. This is because the cycles become very long or very short, as we saw with Catherine's story in Chapter 1. Teenagers may also sometimes experience erratic bleeding as their hormonal cycle establishes itself.

The Pill and Mirena IUS

The hormones in the various formulations of the Pill can often cause irregular bleeding. Women may experience breakthrough bleeding – that is, bleeding between periods – for the first three months or so of starting the combined pill. If it continues, then ask about trying another type. Alternatively, if otherwise things are fine, you may find that you experience breakthrough bleeding if you take the combined pill 'back to back' for more than three months to avoid a bleed. If you're taking the Pill and getting odd bleeding that doesn't settle down, ask about other options or if you need a higher dose.

Irregular bleeding is a common side-effect of the progestogen-only pill, which women who can't take the combined Pill may use. The Mirena IUS also causes erratic bleeding for several months in most women just after it's fitted, but it usually stops after this and then most women end up having no periods.

Pelvic inflammatory disease (PID)

This occurs when an untreated sexually transmitted disease such as chlamydia moves up through the cervix, causing inflammation in the womb, ovaries and fallopian tubes. Symptoms can include bleeding between periods, bleeding after sex, lower abdominal pain and tenderness, painful sex, vaginal discharge, tiredness, as well as fever and nausea. So, if you've got irregular bleeding and these sorts of symptoms and you think there's a chance that you could have an infection (for instance you've had unprotected sex, recently changed partners), it's important to have tests done at a sexual health clinic. It's also a good idea to be screened for sexually transmitted infections before you have an IUD fitted.

A cervical erosion

One of the symptoms of cervical erosion is spotting. This is a harmless condition in which the delicate cells of the inner surface of the cervix start to extend on to the outer part of the cervix in the vagina. These cells bleed more easily after sex, using a tampon or having a smear taken, for instance. It's caused by oestrogen so you may get an erosion if you're on the Pill or during pregnancy or possibly if your cycle is unbalanced in such a way that you are producing too much oestrogen.

An erosion is harmless and usually clears up by itself once you come off the Pill or are no longer pregnant, but, if there's any doubt, your doctor will want to do a smear test. If the cells don't go away and continue to be a nuisance because they cause spotting, they can be cauterized.

An inflamed cervix

If the cervix is inflamed, it may cause bleeding. It's important to find the cause of the inflammation and antibiotics will be needed if there's an infection.

A polyp

A polyp is a small growth on the cervix that is usually painless, but can cause bleeding. If it's a nuisance, it can be surgically removed.

Cervical cancer

This is one of the main reasons doctors are concerned when there is irregular bleeding, as the main symptoms of cervical cancer are abnormal bleeding between periods, after sex or the menopause, as well as persistent vaginal discharge and lower back pain. That's why it's always a good idea to see your doctor if you have odd bleeding. Also, of course, it's important to have your regular cervical smear test.

Cancer of the womb lining

The medical term for this is endometrial cancer. It is more common among older women, from the age of 60s onwards, than it is in younger women. Indeed, it is rare in young women, though the risk starts to increase from the age of about 40.

The symptoms include bleeding between periods or bleeding past the menopause (bleeding more than 12 months after the menopause needs to be investigated; usually there's nothing wrong but about 5 per cent of women will have this cancer), lower abdominal pain, painful sex and tiredness. Risk factors include having a very thick womb lining, being overweight, having too much oestrogen and taking HRT for a long time. Tamoxifen – a drug used to treat breast cancer – may increase risk.

What to do?

If you have unusual bleeding, keep a diary of when it's happening and go to see your doctor.

Tests may include checking the cervix, viewing the womb lining with a hysteroscope, which is inserted through the vagina, and taking a biopsy (a tiny sample of the womb lining) for analysis if it's thicker than normal. Various tests are done to see if the cause is PID, including a cervical swab, a urine test and a pelvic examination.

If there's a problem, the sooner it's treated the better.

Key points

If you've developed abnormal bleeding, don't ignore it. There's usually nothing seriously wrong, but it's best to go and see your doctor about it.

6
Premenstrual syndrome

Many women are all too aware of how premenstrual syndrome – more commonly known by the initials PMS – affects them in the second half of their cycle, but assume that it's a fact of life and nothing can be done about it. Some women don't know what PMS is, but most do, and some dread it because of the way they have been affected by it. Lives can fall apart, relationships break up and jobs can be lost as a result of severe PMS.

Many women feel it's a condition that they have to put up with. They may feel guilty and embarrassed about it or think it's their fault. They fear that they won't be taken seriously if they complain about the problem or they'll be laughed at or that they're imagining the problem – in other words, that they're making a fuss about nothing. Others – particularly younger women who are just starting to get PMS every month – may not be able to put a name yet to these new symptoms they're experiencing. They just feel like life is more difficult at that time of the month. Teenagers may be seen as difficult and moody when, in fact, what they've got is PMS. Sometimes, as Cath explains towards the end of this chapter, it's someone else who puts their finger on the problem – in her case, her mother.

Over the years, Sally realized that she had PMS but she just put up with it.

My PMS crept up on me and became a fact of life when I was in my late thirties. After I ovulated, I felt bloated, my joints were achy and I had a dragging sensation in my lower back. My vagina also felt sore and more sensitive than normal. I was emotionally very touchy and I'd cry at the slightest thing. The world seemed to be against me and I felt everyone was criticizing me, but I never asked for help – I didn't think there was any. Once my period got underway, I felt better, tougher and more able to face the world again.

How common is PMS?

At least one woman in five is affected. According to the National Association for Premenstrual Syndrome (NAPS), around 9 million women in the UK experience PMS symptoms. About 800,000 women are thought to suffer from severe symptoms and a recent study concluded that between about 10 and 21 per cent of women were significantly affected.

What is it?

PMS is a range of physical and mental symptoms that some women feel after ovulation in the second part of their cycle, in the two weeks before their period begins. Once this starts, the symptoms go.

There's a long list of physical symptoms, which include acne, bloating, breast tenderness, changes in bowel habit, nausea, general aches and pains, but especially backache and headaches. Psychological ones include anxiety, feeling low, changed appetite, lethargy, tiredness, mood swings, finding it hard to concentrate and being clumsier and more accident prone.

Some women may suffer from physical symptoms alone, others from emotional and mental symptoms and some from a mix of the two. The severity of symptoms can vary from mild to more severe, while some women may find that their lives are almost unbearable as a result of PMS. A Wellbeing of Women survey of 1500 women found that some women lose 10 days every month as a result of PMS symptoms.

Other conditions and PMS

To make matters worse, other conditions can become more problematic as the levels of the hormones oestrogen and progesterone drop just before a period. For instance, about a third of women who suffer from asthma find that their chest symptoms worsen premenstrually – particularly those with severe asthma. Some migraine sufferers get more attacks premenstrually and some women with epilepsy find that they have more seizures around this time.

Who is most at risk of PMS?

Women aged from 30 to 45 are more likely to have significant PMS symptoms that make everyday life difficult than are younger women. Symptoms can worsen after the hormonal changes that occur, for instance, after childbirth. Indeed, women who suffer from postnatal depression are more susceptible to PMS.

A research study found that overweight women are also more likely to have PMS. It's not yet known what the connection is between this and PMS, though we know that diets full of fats and refined sugars are bad for your health generally.

Research has shown that stress makes matters worse – a finding that is no surprise to Ruth, now in her late forties.

My periods didn't change as the result of having three children, but, after giving birth each time, I developed awful PMS, with bad headaches. Bringing up a family was very stressful and that definitely made my PMS worse. I've noticed that when I'm relaxed and less stressed – for example, when I'm on holiday – I'm much better, perhaps just a bit grumpy.

What causes PMS?

There have been all sorts of theories about why PMS occurs, but what is clear is that it's linked in some way to the hormonal changes that occur in the cycle, as it doesn't happen during pregnancy and stops after the menopause. PMS also seems to run in some families, though no genetic link has been established as yet. Quite what causes PMS is still not fully understood, though it's clear that the symptoms develop after ovulation, in the second part of the cycle, and stop once bleeding begins.

Anxiety and depression, rather than PMS, may be the real reasons behind symptoms for women who complain of problems *throughout* the month – that is, not only in the second but also in the first part of the cycle. One point here – if you feel that your PMS starts early or is unduly prolonged, it is always worth checking with your doctor as to whether or not it really is PMS or relates to some other underlying mental or physical condition. Sometimes, women may blame their symptoms on PMS, but find that their doctors diagnose it as another condition, such as depression or thyroid trouble. As we saw earlier, PMS is related to the ovulatory cycle and, from ovulation to the start of the period is, by definition, 14 days. So, bear in mind that what you are experiencing may not be PMS and, if in doubt, do consult your doctor.

One theory about the link between hormones and PMS that gained acceptance in the past was that women who didn't produce enough progesterone in the second half of their cycles were at risk of PMS. The answer was thought to be progesterone therapy, which was promoted as a PMS treatment. However, that theory has been challenged and progesterone therapy is no longer recommended by many specialists, though it's still available (see below under Medical treatments for moderate to severe PMS).

The current view is that PMS is linked in some way to progesterone production after ovulation, but that it's not insufficient progesterone that is the problem. The answer, according to experts, is that some women may be particularly sensitive to their own naturally produced progesterone because they lack sufficient amounts of a brain chemical called serotonin. This would explain why not all women are affected by PMS. The logical treatment, therefore, is to take an antidepressant that will boost serotonin levels and this option is discussed under the heading Medical treatments for moderate to severe PMS below. Certain foods are thought to increase serotonin levels, so do also look at the section below on diet and try this option first to see if it helps at all.

What helps?

There are now various options on offer, depending on how badly you're affected by PMS. Making lifestyle changes on a number of fronts is often all that's needed to tackle mild to moderate PMS. Supplements may help, too.

The good thing is that, by making these changes, you'll feel more in control of your life, which will reduce stress – one of the possible causes or at least aggravators of symptoms – so this should have a positive effect! If you need additional help, then there are various medical treatments, which are discussed later on in this chapter.

Diagnosis

Keep a diary. This is useful because the first step towards an accurate diagnosis is recognizing what's going on and the easiest way to see this is to analyse a diary recording what happened when over several months. You can chart key information and use this if you need to talk to your GP about getting help. It's a way to take control and make sense of what's happening to you. Looking through your records can clarify whether or not you have PMS in a way that is not possible by just trying to remember what happened. You can see something out of the ordinary is going on if the symptoms persist throughout your whole cycle and not just in the two weeks after ovulation. This could be clinical depression, for example (see under What causes PMS?, above).

The following steps should help if the pattern that emerges from your diary confirms that you have PMS.

Taking control

Diet

Regular meals, eating certain foods and cutting down on others, can make a big difference to PMS symptoms. Helpful hints and tips are given by NAPS, which has a done a lot of work in this area.

What to have plenty of

Eat lots of fruit and vegetables – at the very least five portions a day. Have plenty of fibre and drink lots of liquid (water is best) to reduce the problem of constipation, which affects some women premenstrually.

Carbohydrates are important – particularly the ones that slow digestion and keep blood sugar levels at a steady, optimal level, such as oats, wholegrain breads and basmati rice, rather than ones that cause peaks and troughs, such as sugary snacks.

Starchy foods may improve mood by increasing serotonin levels. It's important – especially during the second part of your cycle – to try and make sure that you have these foods regularly at main meals. In fact, aim to have some starchy food every three hours as snacks. Good snacks include rye crispbread, oatcakes, fruit loaf, malt loaf, dried fruit and low-fat yogurts.

What to cut back on

Go easy on sugar, so watch out for sweets, fizzy drinks, cakes and the like. These sorts of foods will make blood sugar levels go up and down quite quickly, which may leave you feeling snappy and irritable. These foods will also make you feel more bloated.

Salt also increases bloating. Aim to cut back your salt intake to 6 g or less a day – most of us still have far too much, at around 9 g a day. A high-salt diet causes water retention and worsens bloating before your period. There are some simple steps you can take to cut down your salt consumption:

* don't add salt to your food – instead, flavour it with garlic and herbs
* try to avoid smoked or preserved foods, which are high in salt, so, for instance, buy tinned fish preserved in oil rather than brine
* watch out for hidden salt in processed foods and bread.

Be careful, too, about how much alcohol you have. There's evidence that some women use it to cope with premenstrual problems, but it'll make matters worse and could make you more accident prone.

Cut back on caffeine, which may aggravate PMS symptoms and also reduces absorption of various nutrients. The additional benefits from doing this include better sleep and less stress, which, as we've seen, is important. Obvious caffeine culprits are coffee and tea, so try switching to decaffeinated drinks or herbal teas. Watch out, too, for the caffeine you might not expect to find, such as that in fizzy drinks.

Reduce the amount of fat you eat as a high-fat diet may aggravate PMS symptoms. It is wise anyway as such a diet can increase the chances of you suffering other problems, such as obesity, heart disease and cancer.

Exercise

Regular exercise is really important because it's a stressbuster and stress, as we saw earlier, makes PMS worse. Doing something you enjoy and that gets your circulation going will result in the body producing endorphins – the body's own natural painkillers. The upshot is that you'll feel better about yourself as well as fitter. It should also help keep your weight down, which is important as overweight women may be more prone to PMS than slimmer women.

Apart from its well-known general health benefits, exercise can help ease bloating by getting the blood flowing to the pelvis. Some yoga positions can help to combat bloating, indigestion and constipation and the breathing exercises can help you feel calmer, more balanced and stronger. The net result is that yoga helps destress you. However, as with everything, you need to find out whether or not you like it and, if you do, which type of yoga is best for you. Experiment and see what suits you.

Relaxation

Anything that can help you do this is good. Again, yoga is a good way to learn to relax, or you could try tai chi.

Reflexology, which involves massaging and pressing certain points on the soles of the feet, can be beneficial to your health and it is very relaxing. One small study found that it helped sufferers of PMS.

Supplements

Various supplements claim that they're useful in relieving the symptoms of PMS. They may help, but there's conflicting evidence about which ones really are beneficial and some of the supplements are costly. Research results so far suggest that some have more to offer than others, but the picture will continue to unfold as more studies are undertaken. What's needed are results from several large, properly conducted research trials in order to see more clearly what does and doesn't work.

When taking supplements it is important that you don't take more than the recommended dose, unless you are following medical advice. Allow time for it to work, but if you've seen no improvements after about four months, stop taking the supplement.

Vitex agnus castus

Also known as the chaste tree, vitex agnus castus has been shown to be beneficial in a large trial that tried to be as scientific as possible. The study found that agnus castus reduced the severity of symptoms such as low mood, breast pain, headaches and irritability. In the study, 170 women took a daily 20-mg supplement of the herb and reported a significant improvement in their symptoms compared to a group of women taking a placebo (dummy) pill.

There is some evidence to suggest that agnus castus may occasionally make cycles slightly longer or shorter – by, say, a couple of days – but herbalists say that this is nothing to worry about.

Evening primrose oil

Taking a supplement of evening primrose oil is often recommended, but the results of research into its benefits are less definite. It has been found that it helps relieve breast pain, though. However, if you suffer from this symptom you could wear a bra in a larger size during the second half of your cycle, if you find that your size alters then, or else you could try going bra-less as some women find that this helps.

Evening primrose oil contains gamma linolenic acid, which is an essential fatty acid (EFA) and it may be that a lack of EFAs is a cause of PMS.

If you take this supplement, you need to do so for several months at a dose of 240 mg daily to see if it helps.

Vitamin B6

Supplements of vitamin B6 have been reputed to be helpful, but whether or not they really are is unclear at the moment.

Magnesium

This is an important mineral that women often have low levels of and a lack of magnesium may increase the likelihood of PMS. In one study, women who took a daily 200-mg supplement experienced less fluid retention than those taking a dummy pill.

St John's Wort

There is good evidence for the benefits of this herb when used as a treatment for mild to moderate depression and one study found that it helped improve symptoms of PMS. However, if you do decide to try it, check with a pharmacist whether or not it could interact with any other drugs you're taking as it may affect the way they work in the body. For example, it can make the Pill less effective.

Pollen

Pollen may have a role to play in treating PMS. It's early days yet and more research is needed (results of a larger study are due out in 2005), but a small study of 32 women found that those taking the remedy had fewer problems than those on a placebo. 'Femal' can be bought at pharmacies.

Omega 3

These essential fatty acids, found in oily fish such as mackerel and salmon, may help to boost your mood. You can try taking a supplement, but, ideally, eat oily fish regularly instead as it has other benefits to your health, too.

Medical treatments for moderate to severe PMS

It's always a good idea to try the self-help measures outlined above first, but, if these don't work, do get advice about the medical options. Thanks to the pioneering work of gynaecologist Dr Katharina Dalton some 50 years ago, who shed light on what is sometimes a severe illness, PMS is being taken more seriously by doctors.

At one point, progesterone therapy (which was promoted by Dr Dalton) was a commonly used treatment for PMS. As we've seen, the idea behind it was that some women produced too little progesterone in the second half of the cycle so needed a top-up of this hormone. Progesterone and progestogen treatments are still licensed for PMS, but the evidence that they work just isn't there, according to leading PMS specialist Professor Shaughn O'Brien, professor of obstetrics and gynaecology at Keele University School of Medicine, and they may in fact make some women worse. Some studies show that women taking HRT have PMS during the progestogen phase of treatment. According to Professor O'Brien, the treatments that are licensed for PMS don't actually work while those that do aren't licensed for PMS. The other problem, as described earlier, is that it can cause unpleasant side-effects, such as bloating and breast tenderness.

Stopping ovulation

Many doctors say that the way to help women who are badly affected by PMS is to stop ovulation as this does away with the hormonal changes in the second part of the cycle, which, it appears, trigger the problem. This sounds drastic, but may be worth considering if you've tried the lifestyle measures mentioned above and you're still badly affected by PMS. It will, of course, depend on whether or not you want to have a baby and the side-effects of any hormonal treatment you may take.

The Pill

The combined pill – monophasic brands in which the same hormones are taken each day for 21 days, followed by a 7-day break – can help some women. However, others find that this just makes them feel worse because it contains progestogen.

As there are various types of the Pill, it's important to ask which might be the best ones for PMS as they contain different types of progestogen. For example, Yasmin – mentioned in other places in the book – is a relatively new Pill that contains a progestogen that has a mild diuretic effect and is claimed to help those with PMS, though some doctors are sceptical about this claim.

Even though ovulation stops when you're on the Pill, some women still find that they have problems in the Pill-free week because of hormonal fluctuations that may occur then. If that happens, the answer may be to run packs together for up to three months – longer than that and you could get breakthrough bleeding. Ask your doctor about this option.

Mirena IUS

According to one study, having a Mirena fitted may help to alleviate PMS symptoms as it stops ovulation in some women. Also, as the progestogen, which we have seen can cause problems, is delivered locally, such side-effects are less likely to occur. The only thing is that you're likely to experience erratic bleeding for the first few months after having the Mirena fitted, so you have to weigh up all these factors with your doctor and decide what is best for you.

Oestrogen

Some doctors have tried using natural oestrogen, given via skin patches, to relieve PMS. Oestrogen suppresses ovulation, so this may be an option if for some reason you can't take the Pill.

Research shows that this treatment can be very good for severe PMS. However, the downside is that the patches may cause a bit of skin irritation, rashes and possibly some nausea. If you haven't had a hysterectomy, you'll also need to take progestogen in some shape or form to stop the lining of the womb building up too much. However, progestogen may cause PMS symptoms, which would rather negate the point of the patches, so one option might be to have a Mirena fitted.

GnRH drugs

These drugs shut down your monthly cycle, stopping PMS symptoms, but are likely to give you unpleasant temporary menopausal side-effects, so they should only be used in the short term.

It's a complicated business taking these powerful drugs as you'll

89

also need to take some oestrogen to protect against the menopausal side-effects, plus progestogen ('addback therapy', at the lowest possible dose), to prevent the lining of the womb building up. As a result, these drugs are normally used only as a short-term treatment, though specialists may use them for longer.

One 'addback' option might be an HRT product called Livial (tibolone) – a synthetic drug that acts as an oestrogen, androgen and progestogen – though it won't be suitable for all women (as mentioned earlier in the book, there are safety concerns about HRT products – see Chapter 10, the entry regarding safety of medicines in the section under the heading General).

Some doctors use GnRH drugs as a diagnostic tool, to see if a woman really does have PMS. If she does, her symptoms should disappear on this regime because, as you will recall, it's thought that PMS is linked to progesterone production after ovulation, but you don't ovulate when you're on GnRH therapy as your monthly cycle is shut down. If the symptoms persist, however, then doctors are likely to conclude that psychological problems are the real reason for the symptoms.

Danazol

Danazol also suppresses the cycle, but it has unpleasant masculinizing effects and so should only be used for six months.

Topping up serotonin levels

Selective serotonin reuptake inhibitors (SSRIs) are antidepressants that increase serotonin levels. There's some evidence that the brain is less sensitive to progesterone if levels of the brain chemical serotonin are increased.

Prozac is an SSRI that is used to treat severe PMS, though it's currently not licensed for this and it's a question of weighing up the pros and cons of taking this drug, which is more usually used to treat depression. Prozac can help combat PMS symptoms, but there have been concerns that, when it is used to treat depression, SSRIs may make some people feel more suicidal (see the government's Medicines and Healthcare Products Regulatory Agency website to check the latest official advice on this and the NAPS website – both addresses are given in Chapter 10). Obviously the drug is prescribed differently for PMS than depression, in terms of the dosage and length of time you take it for, but ask if this is a concern when it comes to taking it in this way. Ask about its other side-effects, too, as it may occasionally make periods a bit more painful.

This form of drug treatment needs to be tailored to each woman. For example, it can be used continuously, with a lower dose in the first half of the cycle and a higher dose in the second half, or it can be taken just in the second part of the cycle.

Cath says that taking Prozac has made a big difference to her.

My problem started 20 years ago when I was 28, after the birth of one of my sons when I had postnatal depression. Before then I'd had mild problems, which I'd never really noticed. I was probably a bit grumpy, but that was all. Then things got much worse. I became a monster, disagreeable with everyone, got easily upset for no reason and thought that everyone else was at fault. I didn't have any physical problems, but the emotional symptoms got so bad that I parted from my husband for a time. It was my mother in the end who convinced me that I had a problem.

I tried various remedies from the pharmacy, such as magnesium, B6, evening primrose oil and zinc, but nothing helped. I also tried progesterone, but that didn't work either. It was the Prozac that made a big difference. I've been on it for the last ten years or so and if I come off it, my symptoms return. I don't take tablets during my period, then I take one tablet a day in week two, and two tablets a day in weeks three and four.

The Prozac controls my symptoms and I feel more human on it, on an even keel. Without the drug I find it much harder dealing with the world. I keep a diary to keep track of where I am so that I can see when it's my cycle causing problems. PMS has had a huge effect on me and I worry now about whether my teenage daughter will get it.

Key points

Start by keeping a diary so that you can see when your symptoms occur. There are plenty of self-help measures and supplements you can take that should ease symptoms if you do have PMS. There is also a range of medical treatments if you've got moderate to severe PMS. Approaches that work are stopping ovulation or increasing serotonin levels. According to the experts, progesterone therapy is not an effective treatment.

7
Stress control

Stress is a subject that comes up time and again in the context of period problems, which is why this chapter is devoted to it. Women who are stressed may have more problems with PMS and period pain than those who are more relaxed. As a result of stress, periods can become more frequent, heavier or even stop altogether; or you may have irregular bleeding. In fact, cycles can become chaotic as a result of stress, as Lesley found.

> Looking back, I think that stress played a large part in my erratic cycles as I got older. My cycles started to change when I was 38 – partly due to the fact that I was getting older, but also partly due to the fact that I was going through a very difficult time.
>
> My husband and I were trying to start a family, but, when I didn't become pregnant, we went to an infertility clinic. The whole business was really upsetting and I still didn't get pregnant. Then my father died and I remember that my next period after the funeral was much heavier than normal. My mother died a couple of years afterwards, which was really unexpected. My cycles became very short after that for a time – 23-day cycles, then down to 20 days and I began to spot a few days beforehand.
>
> I coped as best as I could, kept a diary and worried. The peculiar cycles continued. I probably did know that I was stressed, but, when you're under so much pressure, you just get through each day as best you can and struggle on.

What is stress?

It's a term we're all very familiar with. It's something to do with feeling overloaded, under too much pressure and finding, as a result, that's it hard to cope with life on a day-to-day basis. You lose that 'mental padding' which helps you cope and bounce back when the going gets tough.

What's stressful for one person may not be for another. We deal with stress in different ways – some people saying that they want and need lots of it and thrive on it, while others are the opposite. Most of us are probably somewhere in between.

In order to understand more about what stress means, we need to look at the stress response, which is the way that we react to and deal with various situations. Current thinking is that it's not events in themselves that cause stress, but, rather, how we see them. The nervous system in the body ensures that vital functions – breathing, digestion and circulation, for example – keep going no matter what. There are two parts to the nervous system. The first is the parasympathetic nervous system, which keeps energy expenditure to a minimum and is calming and relaxing. In contrast, the sympathetic nervous system gears us up to deal with the demands and possible threats that we face each day – it's often called the fight or flight response or stress response.

The adrenal glands – a pair of small glands situated above the kidneys – produce hormones that help us cope when we perceive something as a threat. The part of the gland known as the adrenal medulla produces the hormones noradrenaline and adrenaline. A number of things happen in the body when these hormones are released to get us ready for action. For instance, the pupils in the eyes widen to improve vision, the heart beats faster to pump blood to the brain and muscles, breathing becomes quicker and faster, and blood flow to the skin is reduced because blood is being sent to the legs, arms and main part of the body to prepare it for action.

We need these hormones to get us up in the morning and deal with tasks and if we achieve them we feel good. Good stress – achieving what you set out to do – leaves you with a pleasant feeling of being in control of life and wanting more challenges. It's pressure at its nicest.

However, when we feel that we can't achieve or meet these demands and are overly challenged, the pressure turns to stress. The sympathetic nervous system is switched on for too long and the hormone cortisol is released by another part of the adrenal glands, called the adrenal cortex, to help us cope. The healing parasympathetic system isn't activated enough and the result may be that you feel constantly on edge and threatened. Prolonged chronic stress may affect not only the immune system, making you more prone to infections, but can also disrupt hormones and, thus, the monthly cycle.

The signs and symptoms of stress

Behaviour

You may notice that you're overeating, going for foods you find comforting or, alternatively, you may stop eating. Some people find that they smoke more or drink a lot of alcohol and go in for binge drinking to deaden their senses.

Physical symptoms

These include a fast heartbeat, breathlessness, diarrhoea or constipation, wind, sweaty or cold hands, loss of interest in sex, indigestion, period problems or weight changes.

Mental symptoms

These symptoms include feeling worried, upset, tearful, angry, bored, inadequate, feeling bad about yourself, finding it hard to concentrate and finish a task, feeling woolly-headed, constantly thinking negative thoughts and feeling that the world is against you.

Could stress be to blame?

The first thing to ask yourself is whether or not stress could be responsible for your period problems or making them worse. Recognizing that you're stressed is the first step towards doing something about it.

Taking action

You may be vaguely aware that you're having more problems than normal coping with the world, but spotting the signs and symptoms of stress isn't easy – especially when you're all knotted up! Sometimes it's easier to spot if, for instance, you've suffered a bereavement. Making a connection between the bereavement and how you're feeling and behaving is usually pretty clear-cut. Stress can be harder to spot, though, when it's become long term and you're so stressed that you can't recognize it any more because it is your normal state.

Keeping a diary of how you're behaving and your mental and physical symptoms for a couple of weeks should provide clues to your stress levels. Identifying what may be causing you problems is the next step. Are you exhausted by work and family pressures, do

94

you feel stuck? Can you do anything about the problems you've identified, can you get more help at home if you're struggling to cope with the demands of a family and a job? Unpicking what's behind the stress can be hard, it can take time and it isn't always obvious what you can do about the problem. When it comes to stress there's a useful saying: you should change those things you can and accept those things you can't. Just recognizing you're under stress can also help you to destress!

Your approach to life

Change is an important cause of stress and some of us are better at dealing with it and more resilient to it than others. Dealing with several changes at once, as Lesley had to above, only adds to the problem. Change is part of life, but the pace of change is getting faster and dealing with the adjustments that change requires can be very stressful for some people. There's a long list of stress-inducing life events. Some of those that are particularly stressful are the death of a partner, divorce, separation, illness, marriage, pregnancy, being made redundant, gaining a new member in the family.

There aren't necessarily any quick-fix solutions to any of these sources of stress, but it's true that time is a great healer. Allowing yourself the space and time you need to adjust and being kind to yourself meanwhile will help.

- Time management is important as it'll help to reduce and defuse stress. Prioritize jobs and cut things down to size, breaking up big tasks.
- Keep a narrow focus and don't let yourself be distracted by other thoughts. If you're stressed, you'll find this particularly hard to do, but it means you'll get the job done and that will make you feel better.
- Pace yourself. If something happens that upsets you, allow yourself time to reflect before jumping in straight away with an angry response as this will fire up the stress response.
- Take a break when you feel you're banging your head against a brick wall or that you're about to blow up. If you can, go for a brisk walk and make a big effort to notice what's going on around you as this will widen your horizons. You'll burn off the stress hormones and get your circulation going – all of which should help put life back into perspective again.

95

- Changing how you behave will be a bit stressful, so don't expect it to be plain sailing. Start with realistic aims and expect to feel a bit uncomfortable as you alter familiar ways of doing things.
- Setbacks are normal and not a reason to abandon whatever you're trying to change. Start afresh the following day. Give yourself treats from time to time as a pat on the back!
- Get on with things instead of getting stuck and worrying endlessly about what could go wrong.
- Try something new, even if it seems a tiny thing – doing your normal walking route the other way round, for instance – will help build your confidence.
- Positive thinking will help you to stay cheerful and reduce your anxiety (*No More Anxiety: Be Your Own Anxiety Coach* by Gladeana McMahon, Karnac, 2005) is a useful book on the subject, see Chapter 10 for details). Stressed people usually think very negatively about themselves and the world and these thoughts are usually inaccurate, so challenge them. For instance, the next time you write yourself off, saying, 'I'm a total failure', ask what the evidence for that statement is. You'll find you fail at particular things but not everything!

Other help

Try the following to help you feel more in control.

- Stress dots can start to give you an idea of how you feel when you're stressed. These are dots that change colour as your skin temperature goes up and down. Skin is cooler if you're tense because blood flow is reduced to the skin surface. The opposite happens as you relax. The dot is worn throughout the day on the back of the hand and changes colour according to how relaxed you are.
- Cut back on caffeine, a stimulant. Experiment with herbal teas, such as lemon balm (melissa officinalis), a mood booster, or chamomile, which is calming. Simply add one teaspoon of the dried herb to a cup and pour on boiling water.
- Try plant power. Lavender is well known for its relaxing effects, so put a couple of drops of lavender essential oil in your evening bath for a good night's sleep. Various herbs such as ginseng and rhodiola rosea are powerful stressbusters, but it's best to see a

96

qualified herbalist to be shown how to use them safely. Ginseng, for example, may possibly make periods irregular if taken for more than three months. Other herbs such as St John's Wort may be suggested if you've become a bit depressed. Bach flower remedies such as the rescue remedy can be good if you feel panicky (see Chapter 10 for sources of unformation about herbs and flowers).

- Count how many breaths you take a minute when you're resting. Around 10 to 12 breaths per minute is normal, but 18 or more may mean that you're hyperventilating or overbreathing. Over-breathing is a normal reaction to stress and danger, but breathing should return to its normal pattern once the problem has gone. However, prolonged exposure to stress can lead to chronic overbreathing, which can result in a frightening mix of symptoms, such as a pounding heart, chest-wall pain and tingling in the fingers. Apart from taking a lot of breaths per minute, other warning signs of hyperventilation include yawning and sighing a lot and breathing through an open mouth. Ironically, hyperventilating develops as a response to long-term stress, but it can also increase stress because of all these worrying symptoms that it produces. Physiotherapists who specialize in breathing retraining can teach you how to breathe normally again. In one study of 700 patients, around 70 per cent were cured after treatment and about 25 per cent still developed symptoms when under stress, but could control these by paying attention to how they breathed. To get back to normal breathing, aim for slow, gentle breathing using the diaphragm, the body's breathing muscle below the ribcage. (See Dinah Bradley's book *Hyperventilation Syndrome*, Kyle Cathie, 1991.)
- Get moving! Exercise is great because it burns off stress hormones and also releases endorphins – the body's natural painkillers – and these make you feel good. Do what you find enjoyable, whether it's walking, swimming, dancing, cycling.
- Practise relaxation techniques. There are various types of yoga, but Hatha yoga consists of gentle stretching movements and breathing techniques and so it is especially good for stress reduction. Tai chi is beneficial, too, because it uses breathing techniques together with slow graceful movements that calm you down.
- Have a laugh with a friend. Laughter defuses tension and trusted

friends with whom we can share not only a laugh but also our problems help us cope better with stress.
- A diet rich in B vitamins is good for stress (see the next chapter).

Key points

Stress may well play a part in your period problems, so tackling it should help with these and improve your general well-being.

8
The optimum diet for healthy periods

What and how much you eat and drink has an effect on period health. At its simplest, if you don't eat enough and become very underweight, you may stop having monthly cycles. However, many women these days eat too much of the wrong sorts of foods, become overweight, carry around too much fat and so are at greater risk of developing PCOS, as we saw in Chapter 4. Very overweight women produce more insulin, which may switch on the genes in the ovaries that push up testosterone levels. Fat also produces oestrogen and so may aggravate problems such as fibroids. Carrying around too much weight may also clog up the liver with fat, making it less able to remove excess oestrogen from the body. Being overweight also makes women more likely to get PMS, according to research.

The right diet can keep weight in check, reduce overly high oestrogen levels (linked to conditions such as fibroids, PCOS, painful breasts, cervical erosion, too thick a womb lining) and keep stress at bay – all of which is good news when it comes to period problems.

Taking control of your diet

- Don't make drastic changes overnight because that's not likely to work.
- Don't ban fattening foods you like – instead, have them as occasional treats.
- Downsize portions – we're getting used to supersized ones, with huge plates piled high with food. A normal portion of rice is not five tablespoons, but a couple of tablespoons.
- Allow time – probably several months – for dietary changes to affect cycles. Don't expect period problems to improve overnight.
- Eat a healthy diet all month long and be particularly careful about what you eat in the run-up to your period.
- Eat a wide range of foods to get as many nutrients as possible and use supplements as a backup. If you decide to take one, go for a multivitamin and mineral supplement.

What to eat

If you divide a plate into three, one third should be covered in vegetables or fruit, the second third with carbohydrates and the final third split between high-protein foods, such as fish or meat, low-fat dairy products and small amounts of fat and sugary foods.

Plenty of fruit and vegetables

Have plenty of fresh fruit and vegetables every day – at least five portions, and the more the better. These foods contain a mix of nutrients and chemicals that help to reduce inflammation in the body. They also provide fibre, which will reduce the chances of constipation and help the body to get rid of excess oestrogen in the body. Eat lots of differently coloured fruits and vegetables to get as many nutrients as possible.

Foods such as beans, peas and lentils are excellent because they're low in fat, yet rich in protein and contain two sorts of fibre – insoluble fibre, which helps bowel health, and soluble fibre, which slows digestion and helps to steady blood sugar levels.

Plant oestrogens

Plant oestrogens may also improve menstrual health. These com-pounds, found in vegetables and fruits – particularly soya foods – have a weak oestrogenic effect in the body. They may help by boosting oestrogen levels at the time of the menopause when oestrogen levels are fluctuating and falling. These foods may also help women earlier in their lives by preventing more powerful oestrogenic effects in the body, though this area hasn't been researched in depth yet.

Stable blood sugar

Keeping blood sugar levels on an even keel is important for menstrual health generally, but particularly important if you develop PCOS and PMS.

Eat starchy, complex carbohydrates and whole foods as these are slowly digested, releasing sugars into the blood evenly over a long period of time. Stable blood sugar levels result in less insulin being released. Refined sugars make blood sugar levels go up and down all the time, which encourages insulin to be released to process all that sugar, resulting in cravings when blood sugars are low, which leads

100

to eating more to quell hunger pangs, which leads to weight gain. All this encourages PMS mood swings and PCOS to develop.

The right fats

Fat contains twice as many calories as carbohydrates, so you need to watch your fat intake, though we all need to eat some fat in order for the body to function properly. Fat also produces oestrogen and excess levels of this hormone in the body cause problems, as we've seen.

Unhealthy fats are the saturated ones. Eat sparingly of foods such as butter, hard cheese, cakes, cream, pastries and deep-fried food. Have these as occasional treats rather than every day.

Period pain may be reduced by eating plenty of omega 3 essential fatty acids. Research shows that we don't get enough omega 3 in our diet and have too much of the omega 6 essential fatty acids. Aim to have a diet rich in omega 3 fatty acids, which have an anti-inflammatory effect in the body. The easiest way for the body to access omega 3 in the diet is by eating oily fish, such as mackerel, sardines and salmon, fresh or canned, a couple of times a week. Advice on this may change because of pollution concerns so check the Food Standards Agency website (the address is given in Chapter 10). It's best to get omega 3 from whole foods, but if you can't stomach fish, you may find fish oil supplements more palatable. Other foods to eat include walnuts and sunflower, sesame and pumpkin seeds. Olive oil contains monounsaturated fat, which also has an anti-inflammatory effect in the body.

Support the liver

The liver protects against excess oestrogen accumulating in the body. Help the liver work better by going easy on alcohol and eat foods such as broccoli, globe artichokes, members of the onion family, bitter plants such as dandelion and chicory leaves, as well as pulses, such as peas, beans and lentils.

Keeping your weight in check should also help the liver to work more effectively, as discussed at the beginning of this chapter.

Destress

The B vitamins protect the body from the destructive effects of stress and support the liver. They're found in a wide range of foods, including fish, wholegrain cereals, potatoes, peas, bananas, nuts and green leafy vegetables. Have a bowl of porridge for breakfast as it's a rich source of these vitamins and is non-fattening.

Eat less red meat

We've all been told to cut back on our consumption of red meat for our general health, but it may also be linked to endometriosis.

More research needs to be done into this, but one study found a link between eating red meat and endometriosis. Women who ate seven or more portions of beef or other red meat a week were twice as likely to develop endometriosis as those who ate three portions or less of red meat a week. So, it's a good idea to try white meat instead, such as chicken. Whatever meat you eat, though, make sure to trim off the fat before cooking.

Reduce salt

Having too much salt can aggravate premenstrual bloating, as discussed in Chapter 6. Don't add salt to food and check product labels for salt content when buying food. You will usually find that the sodium content is listed, in which case, multiply the figure by 2.5 to get the salt content.

What to drink

Non-alcoholic drinks

Drink plenty of liquids each day to help your body function properly and stop yourself suffering constipation, as this makes period pain worse. Aim to drink six to eight glasses (ones that are roughly 250 ml/$\frac{1}{2}$ pint size) of non-alcoholic liquids each day. Water is best as it is more readily absorbed and used by the body. Drink more if the weather is hot or you're exercising.

Cranberry juice can help prevent bladder infections, but it also has an anti-oestrogenic effect in the body, may reduce breast pain and possibly help with other problems associated with excess oestrogen. Try drinking 250 millilitres a day.

Soya milk contains plant oestrogens, which, as we saw above, may have a positive role to play in blocking the effects of more powerful oestrogens in the body.

Caffeine

Contained in drinks such as coffee, tea and cola, caffeine is a stimulant that can contribute to stress, may cause breast tenderness in some women and contributes to blood sugar swings, leaving you feeling jittery.

There's evidence that it's addictive, so if you stop straight away, cold turkey style, you may suffer headaches and find it hard to concentrate. It is better to cut down gradually and experiment with having other drinks instead, such as rooibosch tea (red bush tea), other herbal teas and decaffeinated ones.

Alcohol

Treat alcohol with caution and keep consumption to a minimum. Current advice is that it's safe for women to drink up to two or three units of alcohol a day, but not everyone agrees with this.

Alcohol is supposed to have some health benefits because it contains antioxidants, which are good for the heart, but it's not clear exactly how alcohol affects the monthly cycle. At one point it was thought that women were more sensitive to the effects of alcohol just before their period than at other times in the cycle, but this has yet to be confirmed by further research.

What is known is that alcohol is fattening. It's also often described as having empty calories because it doesn't contain nutrients and it may, in fact, reduce the absorption of various nutrients. Women are more quickly affected by alcohol than men as they have more fat and less water in their bodies, which means that women's livers are damaged more quickly by alcohol than are men's. The liver is a vital organ with many functions, including that of getting rid of excess hormones in the body. If it's damaged by alcohol, it can't work so well, which has knock-on effects for other parts of the body.

There's some evidence that women suffering from PMS symptoms may use alcohol to cope with them, but, in fact, doing this can just aggravate problems and make you more accident prone.

Some women may be able to restrict themselves to one or two units a day, but others can't stop at that and may end up binge drinking and getting drunk as a result. It's unclear yet exactly what this does to the monthly cycle, but it's likely to have a disruptive effect.

For all these reasons, it's a good idea to go easy on alcohol and work out ways to reduce consumption. Try having low-alcohol drinks, mix alcohol with water and eat snacks while drinking to slow alcohol absorption.

If you overindulge, remember that alcohol is full of calories, so it will lead to you putting on weight and, if you regularly drink a lot or binge drink, your liver may not be able to work as well as it should, removing less of the excess oestrogen from the body.

Keep an eye on your weight

Before thinking about losing weight, it's important to remember that there are shifts in the fluid content of your body during the monthly cycle. Just before your period, you may find that, temporarily, you're a little heavier than you are the rest of the month.

Body mass index (BMI) and other measures

Finding out your body mass index (BMI) involves doing a few simple calculations and then you can see whether or not you're carrying too much body fat for your own good.

Your BMI is your weight divided by your height squared. A BMI of less than 18.5 means that you are underweight, 18.5–24.9 is a healthy weight, 25–29.9 is overweight and 30 or over is obese, while 35–39 is very obese and 40 or over is extremely obese.

If you don't want to do this calculation, there are various types of body fat monitors that provide information about body weight and composition. There are scales or small, hand-held devices available that do the calculating for you.

A much easier way to keep an eye on your weight is to measure your waist. If the measurement is 81.5–86.5 cm (32–34 in), you're overweight and shouldn't put on any more. If it's over 89 cm (35 in), you definitely need to lose weight and have an increased risk of developing health problems such as diabetes.

So you need to lose weight . . .

If you need to lose weight, don't go on a crash diet as this isn't good for hormonal health. Eat regularly – if you skip meals you're more likely to end up stuffing yourself with high-fat food when the cravings hit as a result of low blood sugar. Eating regular meals is particularly important if you suffer from PMS, as discussed in

Chapter 6. Don't skip breakfast as this can lead to hunger pangs later on. Try a bowl of porridge, which gives you steady supply of energy. Good snacks to banish hunger pangs include fruit – bananas are great for instant energy – low-fat cereal bars, dried fruit and unsalted nuts.

Key points

The monthly cycle is affected by what you eat and drink. A diet that keeps weight in check, reduces excess oestrogen and gives you a wide range of nutrients and anti-inflammatory compounds should reduce period problems.

9

The best exercise

Why exercise?

Many of us aren't physically active and the result is that more and more of us are getting too fat. As we've seen earlier in the book, overweight women have a greater risk of developing PCOS and, of course, other problems, such as diabetes and heart disease. Fatter women are also likely to be producing more oestrogen and too much oestrogen is linked to hormonal problems.

Exercise that gets your heart pumping a bit faster and keeps you physically fit not only reduces your risk of suffering a stroke or developing heart disease or diabetes but also helps promote hormonal health in several ways. It keeps your weight under control, makes your body better able to handle blood sugar so that less insulin is produced (high levels may help trigger PCOS) and exercising reduces the stress that can aggravate period problems.

The body's production of endorphins – the natural 'feel good' painkillers – is greatly increased during exercise and not only helps with pain but also lifts your mood. Getting moving boosts circulation, relaxes muscles, which we tend to tense up when we're stressed and feeling uncomfortable, and all these things work together to reduce the bloating and discomfort that some women experience premenstrually.

What's the best type?

You need to exercise regularly, which means that you need to choose something that's relatively easy to do and will fit into your lifestyle. Better still, choose something you enjoy. People often think of the gym when the word 'exercise' is mentioned. If you like going to the gym that's great, but the problem is that most people don't keep going to the gym in the long term because they get bored with it.

It may not be an obvious choice, but, in fact, one of the safest and most effective ways to exercise to improve not only your general health but also your menstrual health is walking. Large-scale reviews of different exercise programmes have found that walking is the perfect way to get fit because it's easy to do, cheap and can be fitted into everyday life, so you're more likely to keep doing it.

Your walking pace can be adjusted depending on how you're feeling and getting out for a stroll is better than sitting for hours in front of a computer! It doesn't have to be particularly intense for you to benefit a great deal from it. A 30-minute walk that leaves you slightly out of breath – like when you've rushed to avoid being late for an appointment – done five times a week will do you the power of good. Don't overdo it, though, especially if you've got out of the habit of exercising or are very overweight or have asthma or heart problems – if you can't carry on a conversation when you're walking, you're going too fast. Start slowly and then build up to a brisk pace as you feel ready.

Walking is an ideal form of exercise, whatever your age, as it is gentle on the body and unlikely to result in strains and injuries. It's called a low-impact activity because it doesn't put too much stress on your joints or organs so you're very unlikely to hurt yourself.

Getting out into the open, somewhere with some greenery – a park, tree-lined street or the countryside where there are plants and wildlife around you – is even better, as contact with nature has been shown to be a great stressbuster. That's a bonus when it comes to period problems as reducing your stress is important for period health.

If you need to lose weight, a one-hour walk five times a week, going at 4 miles per hour, will burn around 400 calories, which is comparable to a one-hour aerobic class, but a lot gentler on your body.

Build walking into your daily life – the more the better. For example, take the stairs rather than the escalator or lift, choose a shop that's a few streets away to get your newspaper, stretch your legs at lunchtime and pop out for a sandwich, get off the bus one stop earlier and walk home.

One easy way to check how much you're walking is to measure the number of steps you take each day. It's estimated that the average person takes about 3000 steps whereas we should be aiming for at least 10,000 steps a day. It may sound a lot, but it's surprising how they can add up if you take the types of initiatives mentioned above. It's said that doing this should keep you fit and healthy without the need for extra exercise. For more information about this and where to buy pedometers, see the Walking the Way to Health Initiative website (the address can be found in Chapter 10).

Other ways to get fit

It's important to do something that you enjoy because that means you're more likely to stick to it, so if you hate walking but love the gym, do that! Try out other activities, too. You could go for bike rides and/or cycle to work, go swimming or dancing.

Gardening is also great exercise. It's said that tasks such as digging and weeding use as much energy as an aerobic session and being outdoors surrounded by plants reduces stress – and you get a beautiful garden into the bargain!

Exercising safely

If you haven't been very active, build up the amount and type of exercise you do gradually. Before taking a class, make sure that the teacher is professionally qualified. Stop doing anything if it causes pain – the teacher should be able to offer you alternatives that suit you better. If you're doing an intense aerobic class, which puts strain on the body, you should be taught how to do a warm-up first, before you start the exercises, and then a cool-down session afterwards to minimize the chances of injuring your body.

Whatever you do, don't overdo it. Professional dancers and athletes who train really hard can stop having periods and, if that goes on for any length of time, your risk of developing the bone-thinning disease osteoporosis increases. Overdoing it may also lead to the production of the stress hormone cortisol and stop you sleeping at night, which is counterproductive.

When to exercise during the month

Listen to your body, but, as a general rule, do the most strenuous exercising during the middle part of your cycle. One study found that women with regular cycles found exercise easier in the week after ovulation than at the start of their monthly cycles. Exercise more gently in the run-up to your period.

During your period, be guided by what feels comfortable, so, if you feel unwell, stop exercising. At such times you may find the yoga exercises described in Chapter 2 helpful or you could try going for a gentle walk or just rest.

Breathing exercises are a good idea as they should help the womb relax and improve blood flow, which will ease any cramps. This is because our natural reaction when we feel pain is to tense up, but this, ironically, just makes things worse. When muscles are tense, the blood flow is restricted, which causes the pain to increase in a vicious circle. This is why an orgasm can be so helpful as well, relaxing the tense muscles and getting the blood flowing.

To begin breathing exercises, sit down on a comfortable, supportive chair, relax your shoulders down and back, as they are probably tensed up towards your ears if you've been feeling stressed. If they are very tense, try circling them up, back and down or shrugging them right up, taking a deep breath in and then letting them drop as you make a deep sigh out.

When you're ready, breathe in slowly and gently through your nose – filling your tummy with air so it rises and your ribs expand, not just your upper chest – and then breathe out slowly through your nose, making the out-breath longer than the in-breath. (It is important to breathe using your tummy as it helps you to relax and destress fully.) Repeat this. Feel the stress and tension flowing out through your fingers and toes, leaving your body relaxed and calm, yet energized.

Key points

Regular, moderate exercise should improve hormonal health and help weight control, which is also important for the monthly cycle. Don't overdo your exercising, though, as this can stop periods.

10
Where to get more information

Note: If a book is no longer available at book shops, see if your local library has a copy of it.

Acupuncture
British Acupuncture Council
Tel.: 020 8735 0400
Website: www.acupuncture.org.uk

Bleeding disorders (von Willebrand's disease and others)
'A guide for women living with von Willebrand's'
A helpful free booklet available from the Haemophilia Society, which has information about various bleeding disorders.
Tel.: 0800 018 6068 (helpline open Monday to Friday 10 am–4 pm)
Website: www.haemophilia.org.uk

Breathing
Dinah Bradley, *Hyperventilation Syndrome*, Kyle Cathie, 1991

Contraceptives
Family Planning Association
Tel.: 0845 310 1334 (contraceptive education service helpline)
Website: www.fpa.org.uk

Endometriosis
Dian Shepperson Mills and Michael Vernon, *Endometriosis: A Key to Healing through Nutrition*, Element, 1999

SHE Trust (UK)
Tel.: 0870 7743 665
Website: www.shetrust.org.uk

National Endometriosis Society
Tel.: 020 7222 2781
Website: www.endo.org.uk

Epilepsy

Epilepsy Action
Tel.: 0808 800 5050 (helpline)
Website: www.epilepsy.org.uk

Fibroids

Mary-Claire Mason, *Coping with Fibroids*, Sheldon Press, 1997

Website: www.fibroidnetworkonline.com
For general information about fibroids.

Royal Surrey County Hospital
Tel.: 01483 464053
Website: www.fibroids.co.uk
Telephone for more information about uterine embolization.

Website: www.uterine-fibroids.org
For more about focused ultrasound.

Food

Food Standards Agency
Tel.: 020 7276 8000 (UK headquarters' switchboard)
Website: www.food.gov.uk

Glycaemic index (University of Sydney)
Website: www.glycemicindex.com

General sources of information

Kaz Cooke and Ruth Trickey, *Problem Periods: Natural and Medical Solutions*, Allen & Unwin, 2002
Vivienne Parry, *The Truth About Hormones*, Atlantic Books, 2005
Dr Penny Stanway, *The Natural Guide to Women's Health*, Kyle Cathic, 2003

Best Treatments
Tel.: 020 7383 6995
Website: www.besttreatments.co.uk
A useful website that has information on a number of conditions, including heavy periods.

British Liver Trust
Website: www.britishlivertrust.org.uk
For more information about the liver. There is no helpline.

HER (Health Education Research) Trust
Website: www.hertrust.org
This is a new charity concerned with women's reproductive health.

Medicines and Healthcare Products Regulatory Agency
Tel.: 020 7084 2000 (weekdays 9.00 am–5 pm)
Website: www.mhra.gov.uk
For information about the safety of medicines.

NHS Direct
Tel.: 0845 4647
Website: www.nhsdirect.org.uk
A confidential 24-hour service with advice from nurses if you are feeling ill or for health information or contact details of doctors and support groups.

Royal College of Obstetricians and Gynaecologists
Tel.: 020 7772 6200
Website: www.rcog.org.uk
A source of information about women's health, such as the article 'Polycystic ovary syndrome: what it means for your long-term health'.

WellBeing of Women
Tel.: 020 7772 6400
Website: www.wellbeingofwomen.org.uk
A charity promoting women's health that is linked to the Royal College of Obstetricians and Gynaecologists.

Women's Health
Tel.: 0845 125 5254 (health enquiry line)
Website: www.womenshealthlondon.org.uk
Phone the helpline for advice and various leaflets about women's health.

Women's Health Concern
Tel.: 0845 123 2319 (confidential nurse-run helpline)
Website: www.womens-health-concern.org.uk

Heavy periods

Peter O'Donovan with Josephine Waters, *Preserving Your Womb*, Bladon Medical Publishing, 2004

Mooncup
Tel.: 01273 673845
Website: www.mooncup.co.uk
A form of sanitary protection discussed in Chapter 3. The Mooncup is also now available from Boots the Chemists.

Herbs and flowers

Nikki Bradford, *Heal Yourself with Flowers and Other Essences*, Quadrille, 2005

The National Institute of Medical Herbalists
Tel.: 01392 426022
Website: www.nimh.org.uk

Napiers
Tel.: 0131 343 6683
Website: www.napiers.net
A long-established herbal products company. Its creams and so on are widely available by mail order.

Homeopathy

Dr Andrew Lockie and Dr Nicola Geddes, *The Women's Guide to Homeopathy*, Hamish Hamilton, 1992

British Homeopathic Association
Tel.: 0870 444 3950
Website: www.trusthomeopathy.org

Infertility

Infertility Network UK
Tel.: 08701 188088 (advice line Monday, Wednesday and Friday daytime and Monday–Friday 7.30–9.30 pm)
Website: www.infertilitynetworkuk.com

113

Irritable bowel syndrome
IBS Network
Tel.: 0114 272 3253
Website: www.ibsnetwork.org.uk

Menopause
Sally Hope and Margaret Rees, *Managing the Menopause*, Which? Books, 2004

Premature menopause
Daisy Network
Website: www.daisynetwork.org.uk

Miscarriage
Professor Lesley Regan, *What Every Women Needs to Know*, Orion, 2001

PCOS (polycystic ovary syndrome)
Professor Jennie Brand-Miller, Professor Nadir R. Farid and Kate Marsh, *The Low GI Guide to Managing PCOS*, Hodder Mobius, 2005
Christine Craggs-Hinton and Dr Adam Balen, *Coping with Polycystic Ovary Syndrome*, Sheldon Press, 2004
Colette Harris with Dr Adam Carey, *PCOS: A Woman's Guide to Dealing with Polycystic Ovary Syndrome*, Thorsons, 2000
Colette Harris with Theresa Cheung, *The PCOS Diet Book*, Thorsons, 2002
Colette Harris and Theresa Cheung, *PCOS and Your Fertility*, Hay House, 2004

Verity
The Aberdeen Centre
Unit AS20.01
22–24 Highbury Grove
London N5 2EA
Website: www.verity-pcos.org.uk

Verity is a self-help group with lots of helpful information for PCOS sufferers. See the website or send a sae for information (it is hoping to establish a helpline, but regrets that it cannot take telephone calls at present).

PMS

Karen Evennett, *Coping Successfully with PMS*, Sheldon Press, 1995

National Association for Premenstrual Syndrome
Tel.: 0870 777 2177
Website: www.pms.org.uk
Lots of helpful information for PMS sufferers.

Association of Reflexologists
Tel.: 0870 5673320
Website: www.aor.org.uk

Period pain

Neal Barnard, *Foods that Fight Pain*, Bantam, 1999
Susan Lark, *Menstrual Cramps*, Celestial Arts, 1993

Biolamps
Tel.: 0870 240 7097
Website: www.biolamps.com

Ova TensCare
Tel.: 0845 230 4647
Website: www.ova-4u.info
This and various other painkilling appliances are available from pharmacies, but you can buy this direct by phoning the number given above.

Sanitary protection

See the Mooncup under Heavy periods, above.

Sexual health

Mary-Claire Mason, *Sexually Transmitted Infections*, Sheldon Press, 2002

NHS sexual health information
Tel.: 0800 567 123
Website: www.playingsafely.co.uk

Stress

Dr Terry Looker and Dr Olga Gregson, *Stresswise*, Headway 1989
Gladeana McMahon, *No More Anxiety: Be Your Own Anxiety Coach*, Karnac, 2005
Jane Madders, *Stress and Relaxation*, Martin Dunitz, 1981

International Stress Management Association
Tel.: 07000 780 430
Website: www.isma.org.uk

Stresswise
Tel.: 01260 275196
Website: www.stresswise.co.uk
Supplier of stress dots (Biodots).

Thyroid

Patsy Westcott, *The Healthy Thyroid*, Thorsons, 2003

British Thyroid Foundation
Tel.: 01423 709707
Website: www.btf-thyroid.org

Thyroid UK
Website: www.thyroiduk.org

Walking

Dr William Bird and Veronica Reynolds, *Walking for Health*, Carroll & Brown, 2002

Walking the Way to Health Initiative
Tel.: 01242 533258
Website: www.whi.org.uk
For information on how many steps to take each day and how to get a pedometer.

Yoga

British Wheel of Yoga
Tel.: 01529 306851
Website: www.bwy.org.uk

Index

INDEX

exercise 58; benefits of 106; heavy periods and 49–50; pain and 25–6; PMS and 85; stress and 97; types of 106–8; when and how 108–9

fibroids 13, 99; heavy periods 36; medical treatments for 51–4; natural treatments 54; symptoms of 15; types and problems of 50–1
flower essence 22
focused ultrasound 52–3
follicle stimulating hormone (FSH) 4, 73; PCOS and 64
Foods That Fight Pain (Barnard) 24

Geddes, Dr Nicola: *The Women's guide to Homeopathy* (with Lockie) 27
genetic factors 66
gonadotrophin-releasing hormone (GnRH) 4, 29, 54; analogues for heavy periods 44; for PMS 89–90

haemophilia 38
hair, excess 45, 63, 65, 70–1
Harris, Colette: *PCOS Diet Book* (with Cheung) 70
heavy periods (menorrhagia) 20; causes of 35–8; clotting 34; defining 33–5; drug treatments 40–6; medical help 38–41; natural therapies 49–50; surgical treatments 46–9
herbal remedies 26–7; for fibroids 54; for heavy periods 50; for pain 22; for PMS 86–7; for stress 96–7
homeopathy 27, 54
hormone replacement therapy (HRT) 29, 44

hormones: dysfunctional uterine bleeding and 35; heavy periods 37; imbalanced 6, 76; irregular periods 58–60; menstrual cycle 3; monthly cycles 4–5; PCOS 64–5 *see also* individual hormones (e.g. oestrogen)
hot water bottles 21
Hyperventilation Syndrome (Bradley) 97
hysterectomy 33, 48–9

insulin 66, 71, 73–4
intrauterine devices (IUDs) 15–16; heavy periods 36 *see also* Mirena intrauterine system
irregular/missed periods 74; causes and factors of 56–60; spotting between 75–9
irritable bowel syndrome 10, 14

kidney disease 8, 36

Lark, Susan: *Menstrual Cramps* 23
lifestyle: stress and 95–8
liver disorders 8, 36, 101
Lockie, Dr Andrew: *The Women's guide to Homeopathy* (with Geddes) 27
lupus 8, 10
luteinizing hormone (LH) 4, 5, 64

Mason, Mary-Claire: *Coping with Fibroids* 51
massage 23
Mayo Clinic 48
McMahon, Gladeana: *No More Anxiety: Be Your Own Anxiety Coach* 96
medications: aromatase inhibitors 30; for bleeding 38; for endometriosis 29; for heavy

118

(PCOS) 99; becoming pregnant 72–3; diagnosis and treatment 66–72; effects and causes of 62–6; long-term health and 73–4
polyps 36, 78
pregnancy *see* childbearing
premenstrual syndrome (PMS) 13, 99; conditions and causes of 80–2; controlling 84–7; medical treatments for 88–91
Preserving Your Womb (O'Donovan and Waters) 48
progesterone: anti-inflammatory 10; monthly cycle 4–5; ovulation and 12; PMS and 83
progestogen 58; for endometriosis 29; for heavy periods 45–6; Mirena intrauterine system 19–20
prostaglandin 17
Prozac 90–1

relaxation 86, 97
Royal College of Obstetricians and Gynaecologists 39, 45, 54

scans: for adenomysosis 31; investigating bleeding 40; magnetic resonance imaging (MRI) 28, 52–3; polycystic ovary syndrome 66
seratonin 90–1
sex: bleeding after 40, 75; painful 14
smoking 9, 23, 37
sterilization 10, 37
steroids 9
stress 8, 57, 101–2; acting on

94–8; defining 92–3; exercise and 107; pain and 25; symptoms of 94; travel 9

tamoxifen 78
thyroid disorders 6, 7, 8, 40, 59; heavy periods 36; irregular periods 61
tranexamic acid (Cyklokapron) 20, 41–2, 54, 55
transcutaneous electrical nerve stimulation (TENS) 21

uterine embolization 53–4

vitamins and minerals 16–17, 42, 87
vitex agnus castus 86
Von Willebrand's disease 37–8

Waters, Josephine: *Preserving Your Womb* (with O'Donovan) 48
weight factors 8, 57–8, 78; blood loss and 6; body mass index 104; dieting 104–5; PCOS and 66, 67–70
Wellbeing of Women (WOW) 3, 81
womb: cancer of 78; endometrial cancer 70; shedding the lining 4–5, 7; surgical thinning of lining 46–8
The Women's guide to Homeopathy (Lockie and Geddes) 27
Women's Health 34

yoga 23–4